CFRN STUDY G

INTRODUCTION:

Welcome to the Comprehensive CFRN Study Guide: A Complete Review for the Certified Flight Registered Nurse Examination. As a healthcare professional considering a career in critical care transport, you've taken an important step towards expanding your knowledge and skillset. This study guide is designed to help you navigate the challenges of the CFRN examination, providing a thorough review of all the essential topics.

In the chapters that follow, you'll find detailed information on flight and transport fundamentals, respiratory and cardiovascular emergencies, medical and environmental emergencies, and more. Each chapter is organized logically and focuses on key principles that are crucial to understanding and applying in your practice as a flight nurse.

Beyond the technical knowledge, we've also included practical tips for test preparation, study strategies, and a selection of practice questions to help you gauge your progress. By working through each chapter and the practice questions provided, you'll build a solid foundation in critical care transport nursing.

As you embark on this journey, remember that diligence, persistence, and a genuine passion for patient care are the driving forces behind your success. We wish you the best of luck in your pursuit of the CFRN certification and hope that this study guide serves as a valuable companion in your journey.

The CFRN (Certified Flight Registered Nurse) exam is a certification examination for registered nurses who specialize in providing care to patients during air and ground transport. This certification is granted by the Board of Certification for Emergency Nursing (BCEN), a non-profit organization that certifies nurses in various emergency nursing specialties.

The CFRN exam is designed to validate the knowledge and skills of registered nurses who work in critical care transport settings, such as helicopter and fixed-wing aircraft, as well as ground ambulances. The certification demonstrates a nurse's commitment to providing high-quality care in challenging transport environments.

The exam covers a wide range of topics related to critical care transport, including:

General principles of flight nursing, such as safety, transport physiology, and patient management during transport.
Patient assessment and management, including trauma, medical, and environmental emergencies.
Critical care procedures, including airway management, vascular access, and medication administration.
Operational and safety considerations, such as aircraft safety, communication, and disaster management.

To be eligible to take the CFRN exam, candidates must have an unrestricted registered nurse (RN) license and typically need to have experience in critical care or emergency nursing. While not always required, it is highly recommended that candidates have at least two years of experience in flight nursing before taking the exam.

The CFRN exam consists of 180 multiple-choice questions, and candidates are given four hours to complete the test. The passing score is determined using the Angoff method, which involves subject matter experts estimating the difficulty of each question. A candidate's raw score is then compared to the passing standard to determine if they have passed or failed the exam.

Certification is valid for four years, and recertification can be achieved through continuing education or by retaking and passing the CFRN exam.

The exam content is organized into four main content areas, each covering different aspects of flight nursing practice. Here is a more detailed overview of each content area:

1. Flight and Transport Fundamentals (15% of the exam)

This section focuses on the general principles of flight nursing and transport. Topics covered include:

- Transport physiology: Understanding the effects of altitude, temperature, noise, and vibration on the patient's condition during transport.
- Safety and survival: Aircraft and ground vehicle safety, crew resource management, and survival skills in case of an emergency.
- Patient preparation and management: Ensuring appropriate patient preparation and positioning, managing medical equipment, and addressing complications during transport.
- Legal and ethical issues: Understanding the regulatory and ethical aspects of flight nursing, including patient rights and privacy.

2. Respiratory Emergencies (20% of the exam)

This section covers assessment and management of patients with respiratory emergencies. Topics include:

- Airway management: Endotracheal intubation, airway adjuncts, cricothyrotomy, and managing complications.
- Ventilatory support: Mechanical ventilation, non-invasive positive pressure ventilation, and managing ventilator complications.
- Respiratory assessment and management: Recognizing and treating respiratory conditions, such as asthma, COPD, pulmonary embolism, and pneumothorax.

3. Cardiovascular Emergencies (20% of the exam)

This section focuses on the assessment and management of patients with cardiovascular emergencies, including:

- Cardiac assessment and monitoring: Interpreting electrocardiograms (ECGs), hemodynamic monitoring, and managing cardiac emergencies like myocardial infarction, heart failure, and dysrhythmias.
- Vascular access and fluid resuscitation: Peripheral and central venous access, intraosseous access, and fluid therapy in shock and resuscitation.

- Pharmacologic interventions: Administering and managing cardiovascular medications, such as vasopressors, antiarrhythmics, and anticoagulants.

4. Medical, Environmental, and Trauma Emergencies (25% of the exam)

This section covers a wide range of emergencies that flight nurses may encounter during transport. Topics include:

- Medical emergencies: Assessment and management of patients with neurologic, gastrointestinal, renal, endocrine, and infectious emergencies.
- Environmental emergencies: Recognition and treatment of heat and cold-related injuries, altitude sickness, and drowning.
- Trauma emergencies: Management of patients with head, spinal, thoracic, abdominal, and extremity injuries, as well as burn injuries and multiple trauma.

5. Special Populations (15% of the exam)

This section addresses the unique considerations and management of specific patient populations, including:

- Pediatric patients: Pediatric assessment, management of pediatric medical and trauma emergencies, and age-specific interventions.
- Obstetric patients: Assessment and management of normal and complicated pregnancies, labor and delivery, and postpartum complications.
- Neonatal patients: Neonatal resuscitation, assessment, and management of common neonatal conditions.
- Geriatric patients: Recognizing and managing age-related changes and conditions in older adults.

6. Operations (5% of the exam)

This section covers operational and safety aspects of critical care transport, such as:

- Communication: Effective communication with the transport team, medical control, and receiving facilities.
- Disaster management: Recognizing and managing mass casualty incidents and participating in disaster response efforts.
- Quality improvement: Participating in quality assurance and performance improvement activities to enhance patient care and safety.

Exam Eligibility and Application Process for the CFRN.

The examination is administered by the Board of Certification for Emergency Nursing (BCEN). Before applying for the exam, it is essential to understand the eligibility criteria and the application process to ensure a smooth experience.
Exam Eligibility:

To be eligible for the CFRN exam, candidates must meet the following requirements:

1. Active RN License: Candidates must possess an active and unrestricted Registered Nurse (RN) license in the United States or its territories, or the professional, legally recognized equivalent in another country.
2. Clinical Experience: Although there is no minimum clinical experience requirement to sit for the CFRN exam, it is highly recommended that candidates have at least two years of

experience in flight nursing or a related critical care or emergency care setting. This experience will provide the necessary foundation of knowledge and skills needed to successfully prepare for and pass the exam.

Application Process:

1. Online Registration: Visit the BCEN website (https://www.bcen.org/) to create an account and begin the application process. You will be asked to provide personal information, details about your nursing license, and your clinical experience.
2. Application Review: Once you have submitted your application, BCEN will review it to ensure you meet the eligibility requirements. This process typically takes a few business days.
3. Exam Fee Payment: After your application has been approved, you will receive an email with instructions on how to pay the exam fee. As of this writing, the fee for initial certification is $370 for non-ENA members and $230 for Emergency Nurses Association (ENA) members. Please note that fees are subject to change, so always check the BCEN website for the most up-to-date information.
4. Scheduling the Exam: Upon successful payment of the exam fee, you will receive an Authorization to Test (ATT) email containing instructions on how to schedule your exam at a Pearson VUE testing center. The ATT is valid for 90 days from the date of issue, and you must schedule and take your exam within this period.
5. Taking the Exam: Arrive at the testing center on your scheduled exam date with a valid, government-issued photo ID. The CFRN exam consists of 175 multiple-choice questions, with a maximum time allowance of 180 minutes to complete the test.
6. Exam Results: After completing the exam, you will receive a preliminary pass/fail result on the screen. Within a few weeks, BCEN will email you an official score report with your final results.
7. Maintaining Certification: Once you have successfully passed the CFRN exam, you will need to maintain your certification through continuing education and professional development. The CFRN certification is valid for four years, after which you must recertify by either retaking the exam or submitting required continuing education credits.

Test-taking strategies can play a crucial role in achieving success on the CFRN examination. Here are some helpful tips to optimize your performance during the test:

1. Develop a study plan: Create a structured study schedule that allows you to review each content area thoroughly. Set aside dedicated time for studying, reviewing, and practicing each day, and be consistent in your efforts.
2. Focus on your weaknesses: Identify areas where you may need extra practice or reinforcement, and allocate more time to those topics. Use practice questions to identify any gaps in knowledge and adjust your study plan accordingly.
3. Familiarize yourself with the exam format: Understand the structure of the CFRN exam, including the number of questions, question format, and time limit. Knowing what to expect can help alleviate anxiety and increase your confidence on exam day.

4. Practice time management: Develop your ability to pace yourself during the exam. Practice answering questions within the given time frame (approximately 1 minute per question) to ensure you can complete the test within the allotted time.
5. Read questions carefully: Take the time to read each question thoroughly before selecting an answer. Make sure you understand what the question is asking, and eliminate any obviously incorrect choices.
6. Use the process of elimination: If you're unsure of the correct answer, eliminate any options that seem implausible. This narrows down your choices and increases your chances of selecting the correct answer.
7. Answer every question: There is no penalty for guessing on the CFRN exam, so be sure to answer every question, even if you're unsure of the correct response. An educated guess is better than leaving a question blank.
8. Maintain a steady pace: Avoid spending too much time on any single question. If you're struggling with a particular item, make a note of it and move on. You can return to it later if time permits.
9. Stay calm and focused: Remember to relax and stay composed during the exam. Take deep breaths and maintain a positive mindset. Trust in your preparation and knowledge.
10. Review marked questions: If you have time remaining after completing the exam, revisit any questions you marked for review. Double-check your answers and make any necessary changes before submitting your test.

By incorporating these test-taking strategies, you can increase your chances of performing well on the CFRN examination. Remember, thorough preparation, practice, and a focused approach during the exam are key factors in achieving success.

Chapter 1: Flight and Transport Fundamentals

Flight and transport nursing is a specialized field within critical care nursing that focuses on providing high-quality medical care to patients during their transport to healthcare facilities. These patients often require urgent medical attention, and flight nurses play a crucial role in ensuring they receive the necessary care during transportation.

Role of a Flight Nurse in Critical Care Transport

Flight nurses work as part of a dedicated team of healthcare professionals in various transport settings, including air (helicopters and fixed-wing aircraft) and ground (ambulances) transport. Their primary responsibility is to stabilize, monitor, and provide care for critically ill or injured patients during transport. The role of a flight nurse includes:

1. Patient Assessment: Conducting a comprehensive evaluation of the patient's condition upon arrival, including vital signs, medical history, and current symptoms. This assessment helps determine the appropriate course of treatment during transport.

2. Treatment and Intervention: Implementing appropriate medical interventions based on the patient's condition and needs. This may include administering medications, managing airways, and providing advanced life support, among other treatments.

3. Monitoring: Continuously monitoring the patient's vital signs, response to treatment, and overall condition throughout the transport process. Flight nurses must be vigilant and adapt their care approach as needed to ensure the patient's well-being.

4. Communication and Collaboration: Collaborating with other healthcare professionals, such as pilots, paramedics, and physicians, to ensure seamless care during transport. This includes relaying crucial information about the patient's condition and any changes that may occur during the journey.

5. Patient Advocacy: Acting as an advocate for the patient by ensuring their needs are met and their rights are respected during transport. This includes maintaining patient privacy and making informed decisions on their behalf when necessary.

6. Emotional Support: Providing emotional support to patients and their families during a challenging and potentially distressing time. Flight nurses must have excellent interpersonal skills and be able to communicate effectively with individuals from diverse backgrounds.

7. Equipment and Environment Management: Flight nurses must be proficient in using specialized medical equipment found in transport settings and be able to adapt to the unique environment of air and ground transport, such as confined spaces, noise, and vibrations.

8. Continuous Education: Staying up to date with the latest advancements in critical care and transport nursing through ongoing education and professional development. This ensures flight nurses remain knowledgeable and capable of providing the highest level of care to their patients.

In summary, flight and transport nursing is a vital component of critical care medicine. Flight nurses play a significant role in providing expert care to patients during transport, ensuring they reach their destination safely and in the best possible condition. Their unique skillset, adaptability, and commitment to patient care make them an indispensable part of the healthcare team.

Types of Air and Ground Transport

Various types of air and ground transport are utilized to transport patients in need of critical care. Each mode of transportation has its advantages and disadvantages, which are essential to consider when choosing the most appropriate method for a given situation.

Helicopters

Helicopters are a common mode of air transport for critically ill or injured patients. They are highly maneuverable, allowing them to land in tight spaces and reach remote locations quickly. Helicopters are typically used for short to medium distances, making them ideal for situations where time is of the essence.

Advantages:

Rapid response times, allowing for faster access to medical care.
Ability to land in confined spaces or remote locations.
Capable of transporting patients directly to specialized healthcare facilities.
Disadvantages:

Limited capacity, typically accommodating only one patient and a small medical crew.
Susceptible to adverse weather conditions, which can impact flight safety and operations.
Noise and vibrations can create a challenging environment for patient care.
Fixed-Wing Aircraft

Fixed-wing aircraft, such as airplanes, are another mode of air transport used for patient transport. These aircraft are generally reserved for longer distances or when a helicopter is not suitable due to weather or other factors.

Advantages:

Able to cover longer distances at higher speeds compared to helicopters.
Larger capacity, allowing for the transport of multiple patients or more extensive medical equipment.
Generally more stable and comfortable for patients during transport.
Disadvantages:

Requires an airport or airfield for takeoff and landing, which may increase transport time to and from the aircraft.
Less versatile than helicopters in terms of accessing remote or confined locations.
Can be more expensive to operate compared to other transport options.

Ground Ambulances

Ground ambulances are the most commonly used mode of transport for patients requiring medical attention. They are designed to provide a safe and controlled environment for patient care during transportation to a healthcare facility.

Advantages:

Readily available in most urban and rural settings.
Can navigate a wide range of terrain and road conditions.
Generally less expensive to operate compared to air transport.
Disadvantages:

Slower transport times, particularly in heavy traffic or long distances.
Limited in accessing remote locations or areas with poor road infrastructure.
Susceptible to delays due to road conditions, accidents, or other unforeseen circumstances.
In conclusion, each type of air and ground transport has unique advantages and disadvantages that must be considered when deciding on the most appropriate mode of transportation for a specific patient or situation. Factors such as distance, urgency, accessibility, and patient condition should be taken into account to ensure the patient receives the best possible care during transport.

Crew Configuration in Flight and Transport Nursing
The crew configuration in flight and transport nursing can vary depending on the specific needs of the patient and the transport setting. Generally, the team consists of several healthcare professionals who work together to provide the best possible care during transport. The following are common roles and responsibilities of team members in various crew configurations:

1. Flight Nurse: The flight nurse is a registered nurse with advanced training in critical care and transport nursing. Their primary role is to assess, treat, and monitor patients during transport. They are responsible for implementing medical interventions, managing the patient's airway, administering medications, and providing emotional support to patients and their families. Flight nurses also collaborate with other team members to ensure seamless care during transport.

2. Critical Care Paramedic: Critical care paramedics possess advanced training and certifications, allowing them to provide a higher level of care compared to standard paramedics. They work alongside flight nurses to assess and treat patients, administer medications, and manage airways. In some crew configurations, critical care paramedics may serve as the primary medical provider, with the flight nurse in a supportive role.

3. Emergency Medical Technician (EMT): EMTs provide basic life support and assist with patient care during transport. They may help with tasks such as monitoring vital signs, positioning patients, and preparing equipment. EMTs work under the guidance of more experienced medical professionals, such as flight nurses or critical care paramedics.

4. Pilot: The pilot is responsible for safely operating the aircraft during transport. They must have specialized training in flying in various conditions and navigating the specific type of aircraft used for transport, whether it's a helicopter or fixed-wing plane. The pilot also communicates with air traffic control and other relevant parties to coordinate the flight.
5. Respiratory Therapist: In certain cases, a respiratory therapist may be part of the transport team, particularly when transporting patients with complex respiratory needs. Respiratory therapists are skilled in managing mechanical ventilation, providing airway support, and administering respiratory treatments.
6. Physician: While not always present on transport teams, a physician may be included in specific situations that require advanced medical expertise. These physicians are often specialized in emergency medicine, critical care, or a related field.
7. Communication Specialist: A communication specialist is responsible for coordinating the transport mission and maintaining communication between the transport team, dispatch center, and receiving facility. They may provide updates on patient status, estimated arrival times, and any changes in transport plans.

In conclusion, the crew configuration in flight and transport nursing can vary based on the needs of the patient and the resources available. Each team member plays a vital role in ensuring the patient receives high-quality care during transport. By working together and utilizing their unique skills, the transport team can navigate the challenges of providing medical care in a dynamic and often unpredictable environment.

Aeromedical Factors in Flight Nursing

Aeromedical factors significantly impact patient care during air transport. Flight nurses must be aware of these factors and understand how to manage the associated challenges to provide the best possible care. Key aeromedical factors include altitude, cabin pressure, temperature, and others.

Altitude

As the altitude increases, atmospheric pressure decreases. This reduced pressure can cause trapped gases to expand, potentially affecting a patient's condition. For example, patients with pneumothorax or bowel obstruction may experience worsening symptoms at higher altitudes. To manage this challenge, flight nurses should closely monitor patients with conditions that could be impacted by changes in altitude and be prepared to administer appropriate interventions.

Cabin Pressure

The cabin pressure in most medical transport aircraft is maintained at a level equivalent to that found at 8,000 feet above sea level. This reduced pressure can lead to hypoxia in patients, particularly those with compromised respiratory function. Flight nurses must be vigilant in monitoring patients' oxygen levels and may need to administer supplemental oxygen to maintain proper oxygen saturation.

Temperature

Temperature fluctuations can occur during flight, and maintaining a comfortable cabin temperature is crucial for patient comfort and care. Hypothermia or hyperthermia can exacerbate existing medical conditions and complicate patient management. To address this challenge, flight nurses should use blankets or warming devices to maintain appropriate body temperatures and monitor patients for signs of temperature-related distress.

Gas Expansion

Changes in cabin pressure can lead to the expansion of gases within body cavities or medical equipment, such as intravenous (IV) bags and endotracheal tubes. Flight nurses must be aware of these potential issues and take steps to minimize their impact, such as venting IV bags or adjusting the pressure settings on medical devices.

Vibration and Noise

Vibration and noise are inherent in air transport and can affect both patients and medical crew members. These factors can cause fatigue, disorientation, and difficulty communicating, making it challenging to provide optimal patient care. Flight nurses can manage these issues by using noise-reduction headsets, minimizing unnecessary conversation, and securing equipment to reduce vibrations.

In conclusion, aeromedical factors play a significant role in flight nursing and patient care during air transport. By understanding these factors and implementing strategies to address the challenges they pose, flight nurses can ensure the safe and effective care of patients throughout the transport process.

Communication and Coordination in Transport Nursing
Effective communication and teamwork are vital to ensuring the success of patient transport in flight and ground nursing. This involves coordination among crew members, the dispatch center, and receiving facilities. Let's explore the importance of communication and teamwork, along with strategies to overcome potential communication barriers.
Importance of Effective Communication
1. Patient Safety: Clear and accurate communication among team members helps ensure patient safety by facilitating a seamless handoff of care, preventing medical errors, and enabling efficient problem-solving during emergencies.
2. Timely Care Delivery: Effective communication between the transport team and receiving facilities allows for proper preparation and patient care coordination. This ensures that essential resources and personnel are ready upon the patient's arrival.

3. Crew Resource Management: Efficient teamwork and communication among crew members allow each person to contribute their expertise effectively, leading to better decision-making and resource utilization.
4. Situation Awareness: Regular updates on the patient's condition and progress during transport keep all parties informed and help maintain a shared understanding of the situation, enabling a more effective response to any changes.

Methods for Overcoming Communication Barriers

1. Standardized Language and Terminology: Using standardized language and medical terminology helps prevent misunderstandings and misinterpretations. All team members should be familiar with common abbreviations, acronyms, and terms used in transport nursing.
2. Closed-Loop Communication: This technique involves repeating back critical information to ensure accurate understanding. For example, when a flight nurse receives an instruction from a colleague, they should repeat the instruction to confirm they understood it correctly.
3. Communication Aids: Tools like noise-cancelling headsets, hand signals, and written communication can help overcome the challenges of noisy or chaotic environments. These aids facilitate clear communication between team members during transport.
4. Briefings and Debriefings: Regular briefings before and after transport missions help establish a shared understanding of the patient's condition, the plan of care, and any potential challenges. Debriefings offer an opportunity to review the transport and identify areas for improvement.
5. Training and Simulation: Participating in communication and teamwork training, including simulation exercises, can help transport nursing personnel develop and hone their skills. These exercises provide a safe environment to practice effective communication techniques and learn from potential mistakes.

In conclusion, effective communication and teamwork are essential components of successful patient transport in flight and ground nursing. By focusing on clear and accurate communication, utilizing various tools and techniques, and participating in regular training, transport nursing teams can overcome potential barriers and ensure the highest quality of care for their patients.

Patient Safety and Risk Management

Ensuring patient safety and minimizing risks during flight and ground transport are of utmost importance. Various safety measures, equipment, and protocols can help maintain a secure transport environment. Crew members play a crucial role in adhering to these guidelines and fostering a culture of safety.

Essential Safety Measures

1. Pre-transport Assessment: Before transport, evaluate the patient's condition, review medical records, and identify any potential risks or special needs. Ensure that the patient is stable enough for transport and determine the appropriate level of care required during the journey.

2. Equipment Safety: Inspect and maintain all medical and safety equipment regularly to ensure proper functioning. Verify that devices are calibrated and have adequate power sources. Secure equipment and supplies to prevent movement during transport.
3. Crew Training and Competency: Regularly participate in ongoing training and skill development to maintain proficiency in emergency procedures, equipment use, and patient care. This ensures that crew members can effectively respond to any situation that may arise during transport.
4. Infection Control: Adhere to infection control protocols, including hand hygiene, use of personal protective equipment (PPE), and proper cleaning and disinfection of equipment and surfaces. This helps prevent the spread of infections among patients and crew members.
5. Communication and Coordination: Maintain open lines of communication with the transport team, dispatch center, and receiving facility. Share critical information and updates regarding the patient's condition, potential risks, and the estimated time of arrival.

Crew Members' Responsibilities
1. Vigilance and Monitoring: Continuously monitor the patient's vital signs, symptoms, and response to interventions during transport. Be prepared to respond to any changes in the patient's condition or unexpected events that may occur.
2. Medication Safety: Administer medications accurately and safely, following the "five rights" of medication administration: right patient, right medication, right dose, right route, and right time. Double-check medications, doses, and infusion rates with another crew member when possible.
3. Adherence to Protocols and Guidelines: Follow established protocols and guidelines for patient care, equipment use, and emergency procedures. This ensures consistent and high-quality care across the transport team.
4. Reporting and Documentation: Accurately document all aspects of patient care during transport, including assessments, interventions, and patient responses. Report any incidents or near misses to promote learning and continuous improvement.
5. Promote a Culture of Safety: Actively participate in safety initiatives, debriefings, and quality improvement efforts. Encourage open communication and constructive feedback within the transport team to identify and address potential risks and areas for improvement.

In summary, patient safety and risk management are essential aspects of flight and ground transport nursing. By implementing safety measures, adhering to protocols, and fostering a culture of safety, transport nursing teams can minimize risks and ensure the highest level of care for their patients.

In-Flight Medical Emergencies
Flight and transport nurses may encounter various medical emergencies during patient transport. Understanding the common scenarios and the appropriate assessment, intervention, and management strategies is vital for providing the best possible care. Here, we discuss some common in-flight medical emergencies and their respective management strategies.
1. Respiratory Distress

Respiratory distress can result from various conditions, including asthma, chronic obstructive pulmonary disease (COPD), or pneumonia. Key management strategies include:

- Assess and monitor the patient's respiratory rate, oxygen saturation, and lung sounds.
- Administer supplemental oxygen and ensure a patent airway.
- Administer medications such as bronchodilators or corticosteroids, if indicated.
- Monitor the patient's response to interventions and adjust treatment as needed.

2. Cardiovascular Emergencies

Cardiovascular emergencies, such as acute myocardial infarction or congestive heart failure, require rapid assessment and intervention. Key management strategies include:

- Continuously monitor vital signs, including heart rate, blood pressure, and cardiac rhythm.
- Administer supplemental oxygen to maintain adequate oxygen saturation.
- Administer medications such as nitrates, beta-blockers, or diuretics, if indicated.
- Notify the receiving facility of the patient's condition and prepare for potential advanced cardiac interventions.

3. Seizures

Seizures can occur due to epilepsy, brain injury, or other neurological disorders. Key management strategies include:

- Protect the patient from injury by providing a safe environment.
- Monitor the patient's airway, breathing, and vital signs.
- Administer anticonvulsant medications, if indicated and prescribed.
- Assess for potential underlying causes, such as hypoglycemia, and address them accordingly.

4. Hypoglycemia

Hypoglycemia can result from various factors, including insulin overdose or inadequate food intake in diabetic patients. Key management strategies include:

- Assess the patient's blood glucose level and mental status.
- Administer oral or intravenous glucose, depending on the patient's level of consciousness and ability to swallow.
- Monitor the patient's response to treatment and recheck blood glucose levels as needed.
- Notify the receiving facility of the patient's condition and any interventions provided.

5. Trauma-Related Emergencies

Trauma-related emergencies can result from motor vehicle accidents, falls, or other incidents leading to injuries. Key management strategies include:

- Assess the patient's airway, breathing, and circulation using the primary survey (ABCDE).
- Stabilize and immobilize fractures, dislocations, or other injuries as needed.
- Control bleeding using direct pressure, elevation, or tourniquet application, if indicated.
- Continuously monitor vital signs and neurological status.

In summary, flight and transport nurses must be prepared to handle a variety of medical emergencies. By understanding the appropriate assessment, intervention, and management strategies for each scenario, nurses can provide timely and effective care to patients during flight and transport.

Transport Equipment and Technology

Flight and transport nurses utilize a range of specialized equipment and technology to provide high-quality care during patient transport. Understanding the function and proper use of these tools is essential to ensure patient safety and optimal outcomes. In this section, we'll explore various types of equipment and technology commonly used in transport nursing, as well as the importance of equipment maintenance and troubleshooting.

Ventilators
Ventilators are essential for patients requiring respiratory support during transport. Transport ventilators are often portable and designed to withstand the unique challenges of flight and ground transport, such as changes in cabin pressure and temperature. Nurses must be proficient in ventilator settings, adjustments, and troubleshooting to provide optimal care for patients with respiratory needs.

Monitors
Patient monitoring is critical during transport to ensure timely identification and intervention for any clinical changes. Transport monitors are typically compact, portable, and designed to provide continuous data on vital signs, cardiac rhythms, oxygen saturation, and end-tidal CO_2 levels. Nurses must be familiar with the use and interpretation of monitor data to guide patient care decisions.

Infusion Devices
Infusion devices, such as infusion pumps or syringe pumps, are used to deliver medications, fluids, and blood products at precise rates during transport. Transport nurses must understand the proper setup, programming, and troubleshooting of these devices to ensure safe and accurate medication administration.

Airway Management Tools
Airway management tools, including laryngoscopes, endotracheal tubes, and supraglottic airways, are crucial for establishing and maintaining a patent airway during transport. Nurses must be proficient in the use of these tools and the appropriate techniques for airway management, including intubation and ventilation.

Defibrillators
Defibrillators are vital for managing cardiac emergencies during transport. Transport defibrillators are often lightweight and portable, with both manual and automated external defibrillator (AED) capabilities. Nurses must be familiar with the operation of these devices and the appropriate treatment protocols for various cardiac arrhythmias.

Equipment Maintenance and Troubleshooting

Proper equipment maintenance and troubleshooting are essential to ensure patient safety and minimize the risk of equipment-related complications during transport. Regular inspection, cleaning, and calibration of equipment are crucial to maintain optimal function. Nurses must also be knowledgeable about the common issues and troubleshooting techniques for each device, such as battery replacements, alarm management, and error code resolution.

In summary, transport equipment and technology are critical components of patient care during flight and ground transport. Flight and transport nurses must be well-versed in the use, maintenance, and troubleshooting of various devices to provide safe and effective care to their patients.

Chapter 2: Respiratory Emergencies

Respiratory distress can be a life-threatening condition that requires prompt identification and intervention. Recognizing the signs and symptoms early, as well as understanding the steps for assessment and management, is crucial in providing effective care during patient transport. Signs and symptoms of respiratory distress include increased respiratory rate (tachypnea), shortness of breath (dyspnea), use of accessory muscles, nasal flaring, intercostal retractions, cyanosis, and altered mental status. Early recognition is vital as it allows for timely intervention, preventing potential complications, and ensuring the patient's safety during transport.

To assess and manage a patient experiencing respiratory distress during transport, follow these steps:

1. Assess the airway: Ensure the patient's airway is patent and free of any obstructions. If necessary, reposition the head or use airway adjuncts, such as oral or nasal airways.
2. Evaluate breathing: Assess the patient's respiratory rate, depth, and pattern. Auscultate lung sounds and observe chest movement for symmetry. Be attentive to any signs of labored breathing or difficulty in maintaining airway patency.
3. Administer oxygen: Provide supplemental oxygen, if required, based on the patient's oxygen saturation levels and clinical presentation. Adjust the oxygen delivery method and flow rate as needed to maintain appropriate oxygenation.
4. Monitor vital signs: Continuously monitor the patient's heart rate, blood pressure, respiratory rate, oxygen saturation, and level of consciousness. Look for any changes that may indicate worsening respiratory distress or the need for further intervention.
5. Provide pharmacological interventions: Depending on the cause of respiratory distress, administer medications as indicated, such as bronchodilators for asthma, diuretics for congestive heart failure, or corticosteroids for inflammation.
6. Consider advanced airway management: If the patient's condition deteriorates or fails to improve with initial interventions, consider advanced airway management techniques, such as non-invasive ventilation (e.g., continuous positive airway pressure (CPAP) or bilevel positive airway pressure (BiPAP)) or endotracheal intubation.
7. Reassess and reevaluate: Regularly reassess the patient's response to interventions, adjust treatments as necessary, and communicate any changes in the patient's condition to the receiving facility.

By understanding the signs and symptoms of respiratory distress and the steps involved in assessing and managing a patient experiencing this condition during transport, you can provide effective care and ensure the best possible outcome for your patient.

Airway obstruction can be a life-threatening emergency that demands rapid identification and intervention. Recognizing the various causes, understanding the clinical presentation, and knowing the appropriate management techniques are essential skills for effectively addressing airway obstructions during patient transport.

Causes of airway obstruction can be broadly classified into three categories:

1. Mechanical: Foreign body aspiration, trauma, swelling, or masses in the airway.

2. Functional: Decreased muscle tone or neurological impairment affecting airway patency, such as in sedated patients or those with neuromuscular disorders.
3. Inflammatory: Infections, allergic reactions, or inflammation causing airway narrowing or swelling.

Clinical presentation of a patient with an obstructed airway may include:
- Difficulty breathing or inability to speak
- Stridor (high-pitched, noisy breathing) or wheezing
- Use of accessory muscles or retractions
- Cyanosis (bluish discoloration of the skin)
- Altered mental status or agitation

To manage airway obstruction during patient transport, consider the following interventions:
1. Positioning: Place the patient in a position that optimizes airway patency, such as a head-tilt, chin-lift, or jaw-thrust maneuver, depending on the patient's level of consciousness and suspected cause of obstruction.
2. Suctioning: Use a portable suction device to remove secretions, blood, or vomitus from the airway, as needed.
3. Airway adjuncts: If the patient's airway remains obstructed or compromised, insert an oral or nasal airway to help maintain patency.
4. Manual removal: For a visible foreign body obstruction, attempt manual removal using a finger sweep or Magill forceps.
5. Advanced airway management: If the patient's airway remains obstructed despite basic interventions, consider advanced airway techniques, such as endotracheal intubation, supraglottic airway devices, or needle cricothyrotomy.
6. Monitor and reassess: Continuously monitor the patient's vital signs, oxygen saturation, and respiratory status. Reassess the effectiveness of interventions and adjust as necessary.
7. Communicate: Keep the receiving facility informed of the patient's condition, interventions performed, and any changes in their status.

By understanding the causes, clinical presentation, and management of airway obstruction during patient transport, you can provide appropriate and timely care, ensuring the best possible outcome for your patient.

Mechanical ventilation is a crucial aspect of managing patients with respiratory compromise during transport. Understanding the principles, modes, and settings, as well as the importance of monitoring and adjusting the ventilator, is essential for optimal patient care.

Principles of mechanical ventilation involve delivering a set volume or pressure of air to the patient's lungs to support or replace their natural breathing. The primary goals are to ensure adequate oxygenation, facilitate carbon dioxide removal, and minimize lung injury.

There are several modes of mechanical ventilation commonly used in transport:
1. Volume-Controlled Ventilation (VCV): This mode delivers a predetermined tidal volume (VT) to the patient, regardless of the pressure required. It's often used for patients with healthy lungs who need temporary ventilatory support.

2. Pressure-Controlled Ventilation (PCV): The ventilator delivers a set pressure, and the tidal volume varies depending on the patient's lung compliance. PCV is often preferred for patients with acute lung injury or acute respiratory distress syndrome (ARDS).
3. Synchronized Intermittent Mandatory Ventilation (SIMV): This mode combines controlled breaths with the patient's spontaneous breaths, synchronizing the ventilator-delivered breaths with the patient's natural breathing efforts.
4. Pressure Support Ventilation (PSV): This mode provides a set pressure during spontaneous breaths, supporting the patient's effort to overcome airway resistance and reducing the work of breathing.

Key ventilator settings to be aware of include:
- Tidal Volume (VT): The volume of air delivered with each breath, typically set at 6-8 mL/kg of ideal body weight.
- Respiratory Rate (RR): The number of breaths per minute, adjusted based on the patient's needs and blood gas analysis.
- Inspiratory to Expiratory (I:E) ratio: The ratio of time spent in inspiration to expiration, usually set at 1:2 for most patients.
- Positive End-Expiratory Pressure (PEEP): A continuous pressure applied at the end of expiration to maintain alveolar recruitment and prevent lung collapse.
- Fraction of Inspired Oxygen (FiO2): The concentration of oxygen being delivered, adjusted to maintain adequate oxygenation without causing hyperoxia.

Monitoring and adjusting ventilator settings during transport are critical for ensuring patient safety and optimizing care. Pay close attention to:
- Vital signs: Continuously monitor heart rate, blood pressure, and oxygen saturation.
- Breath sounds: Assess lung sounds frequently to evaluate ventilation and detect complications.
- Ventilator alarms: Respond promptly to alarms indicating high pressure, low pressure, or apnea.
- Blood gas analysis: Obtain arterial blood gas samples to assess oxygenation, ventilation, and acid-base balance.

By understanding the principles, modes, and settings of mechanical ventilation, as well as the importance of monitoring and adjusting the ventilator during transport, you can provide the best possible care for patients requiring ventilatory support.

Specific Respiratory Emergencies.

Acute respiratory failure is a life-threatening condition where the respiratory system fails to maintain adequate gas exchange, leading to hypoxia, hypercapnia, or both. Understanding the causes, clinical manifestations, and management strategies is crucial for providing appropriate care during patient transport.

Causes of acute respiratory failure can be divided into two main categories:
1. Type I (hypoxemic) respiratory failure, where the primary issue is oxygenation. Common causes include pneumonia, acute respiratory distress syndrome (ARDS), pulmonary edema, and pulmonary embolism.

2. Type II (hypercapnic) respiratory failure, where the primary issue is ventilation. Causes may include neuromuscular disorders, chronic obstructive pulmonary disease (COPD), obesity hypoventilation syndrome, and chest wall deformities.

Clinical manifestations of acute respiratory failure include:

- Dyspnea (shortness of breath)
- Tachypnea (increased respiratory rate)
- Cyanosis (bluish discoloration of the skin)
- Altered mental status
- Accessory muscle use
- Hypoxia or hypercapnia as evidenced by blood gas analysis

Management strategies for acute respiratory failure during transport involve a stepwise approach:

1. Supplemental oxygen: Provide oxygen via nasal cannula, simple face mask, or non-rebreather mask, titrating the flow rate to maintain adequate oxygen saturation (typically above 90%).
2. Non-invasive ventilation (NIV): Consider using continuous positive airway pressure (CPAP) or bilevel positive airway pressure (BiPAP) for patients with moderate to severe respiratory distress who are able to protect their airway. NIV is particularly useful for patients with COPD exacerbations, cardiogenic pulmonary edema, and some cases of ARDS.
3. Invasive ventilation: Intubation and mechanical ventilation may be necessary for patients with severe respiratory failure who are unable to maintain adequate oxygenation or ventilation, exhibit a deteriorating mental status, or have failed NIV. Follow the principles and modes of mechanical ventilation as described in previous sections, and closely monitor the patient's vital signs, breath sounds, and blood gases.

Chapter 3: Cardiovascular Emergencies

The Cardiovascular Emergencies chapter focuses on the recognition, assessment, and management of various life-threatening conditions affecting the heart and circulatory system during patient transport. Key subjects covered in this chapter include:

1. Chest Pain: Understanding the various causes of chest pain, such as acute coronary syndromes, aortic dissection, pulmonary embolism, and non-cardiac etiologies, as well as the importance of early recognition and appropriate management, including ECG monitoring and pharmacological interventions.
2. Acute Coronary Syndromes (ACS): Exploring the pathophysiology, presentation, and management of unstable angina, NSTEMI, and STEMI, with emphasis on the role of ECG interpretation, antiplatelet and anticoagulant therapy, and timely reperfusion strategies.
3. Heart Failure and Pulmonary Edema: Discussing the pathophysiology, clinical manifestations, and management of acute heart failure and pulmonary edema during transport, including the use of oxygen therapy, diuretics, vasodilators, and inotropes.
4. Cardiac Arrhythmias: Examining various types of arrhythmias, such as atrial fibrillation, ventricular tachycardia, and ventricular fibrillation, as well as their potential impact on hemodynamic stability, and the appropriate pharmacological and electrical therapies for each condition.
5. Cardiogenic Shock: Understanding the causes, clinical presentation, and management of cardiogenic shock, focusing on the importance of early recognition, aggressive hemodynamic support, and definitive interventions to restore cardiac function and perfusion.

Throughout the chapter, emphasis is placed on the importance of rapid assessment, timely interventions, and ongoing monitoring of patients experiencing cardiovascular emergencies during transport. The goal is to provide transport nurses and other healthcare professionals with the knowledge and skills necessary to deliver optimal care and improve patient outcomes in these critical situations.

Chest pain is a concerning symptom that may indicate a variety of underlying conditions, some of which can be life-threatening. Early recognition and appropriate management of chest pain during patient transport are crucial for achieving the best possible outcomes.

There are numerous potential causes of chest pain, including cardiac, pulmonary, gastrointestinal, and musculoskeletal issues. Cardiac causes, such as acute coronary syndromes (unstable angina, NSTEMI, and STEMI), are of particular concern due to their potential for severe complications and death. Other cardiac causes include pericarditis, myocarditis, and aortic dissection. Pulmonary causes include pulmonary embolism, pneumothorax, and pleurisy. Gastrointestinal causes, such as gastroesophageal reflux disease (GERD) and esophageal spasm, can also mimic cardiac chest pain. Musculoskeletal causes, like costochondritis, are usually less severe but can still cause significant discomfort.

To effectively manage chest pain during transport, the first step is conducting a thorough patient assessment. This includes obtaining a detailed history, including the nature, location, and duration of the pain, as well as any associated symptoms, such as shortness of breath, nausea, or diaphoresis. Vital signs should be monitored closely, and a physical examination should be performed to identify any abnormalities.

ECG monitoring is an essential component of the assessment process. A 12-lead ECG can help identify potential cardiac causes of chest pain, such as acute coronary syndromes or arrhythmias, and guide treatment decisions. Serial ECGs may be needed to detect evolving changes, especially in the case of acute coronary syndromes.

Pharmacological interventions are an important aspect of managing chest pain during transport. For suspected cardiac chest pain, medications such as aspirin, nitroglycerin, and opioids (e.g., morphine) may be administered to alleviate pain and reduce the workload on the heart. Oxygen therapy should be provided as needed, based on the patient's oxygen saturation and clinical condition. In cases of arrhythmias, antiarrhythmic medications or electrical therapy, such as defibrillation or cardioversion, may be necessary.

In summary, effective assessment and management of chest pain during patient transport are essential for ensuring optimal patient outcomes. Identifying the underlying cause, closely monitoring the patient's condition, and administering appropriate pharmacological and non-pharmacological interventions can significantly impact the patient's prognosis.

Acute Coronary Syndromes (ACS) are a spectrum of conditions resulting from decreased blood flow to the heart muscle, typically caused by a rupture or erosion of an atherosclerotic plaque in the coronary arteries. ACS encompasses unstable angina (UA), non-ST elevation myocardial infarction (NSTEMI), and ST-elevation myocardial infarction (STEMI).

Pathophysiology: ACS is primarily caused by the formation of a blood clot (thrombus) in response to a damaged coronary artery, impeding blood flow to the heart muscle. The degree of artery blockage and duration of reduced blood flow dictate the severity and type of ACS. Unstable angina occurs when the thrombus is only partially occlusive, while NSTEMI and STEMI occur when the thrombus is more significant, causing damage to the heart muscle.

Clinical Presentation: Patients with ACS often present with chest pain or discomfort, which may radiate to the arms, neck, jaw, or back. Associated symptoms can include shortness of breath, sweating, nausea, vomiting, lightheadedness, and palpitations. In some cases, symptoms may be atypical or absent, particularly in women, elderly patients, and those with diabetes.

Management: Early recognition and intervention are crucial in ACS management. In the prehospital setting, healthcare providers should obtain a 12-lead electrocardiogram (ECG) to differentiate between unstable angina, NSTEMI, and STEMI. Aspirin should be administered as soon as possible, and nitroglycerin may be given for ongoing chest pain.

For NSTEMI and unstable angina, anticoagulants such as heparin, along with antiplatelet agents like clopidogrel, are typically administered. Depending on the patient's risk profile and the availability of specialized cardiac care, invasive strategies such as cardiac catheterization and percutaneous coronary intervention (PCI) may be pursued.

In STEMI, the primary goal is to restore blood flow to the affected heart muscle as quickly as possible, ideally through PCI at a specialized cardiac care facility. If PCI is not available within the recommended timeframe, fibrinolytic therapy (clot-busting medication) should be considered.

Coordination with Receiving Facilities: Effective communication and coordination between prehospital providers and receiving facilities are essential to minimize delays and ensure timely intervention. This includes promptly transmitting ECG findings, alerting the receiving facility of a potential ACS patient, and activating the cardiac catheterization laboratory if needed.

Overall, understanding the pathophysiology, clinical presentation, and management of ACS is vital for transport nurses and other healthcare professionals to provide optimal care and improve patient outcomes in these critical situations.

Heart failure and cardiogenic shock are severe cardiovascular emergencies that require prompt recognition and management during patient transport. In heart failure, the heart is unable to pump blood effectively, while cardiogenic shock is a more critical condition in which the heart is unable to provide adequate blood flow to meet the body's needs.

Causes: Heart failure can be caused by several factors, including coronary artery disease, hypertension, valvular heart disease, and cardiomyopathies. Cardiogenic shock often occurs as a complication of a severe heart attack or worsening heart failure.

Clinical Manifestations: Patients with heart failure may present with shortness of breath, fatigue, fluid retention, and pulmonary edema. In cardiogenic shock, the clinical presentation may include hypotension, altered mental status, weak or absent peripheral pulses, cold and clammy skin, and oliguria (low urine output).

Management Strategies: In the transport setting, management of heart failure and cardiogenic shock focuses on stabilizing the patient and initiating appropriate interventions.

Pharmacological agents play a significant role in managing these conditions. In heart failure, medications such as diuretics, vasodilators, and inotropic agents may be used to alleviate symptoms and improve cardiac function. In cardiogenic shock, vasopressors and inotropic agents are often necessary to maintain blood pressure and support cardiac output.

Mechanical circulatory support devices, such as intra-aortic balloon pumps (IABP) or ventricular assist devices (VAD), may be utilized in severe cases of cardiogenic shock. These devices help improve blood flow and maintain organ perfusion while the underlying cause of the shock is being treated.

Collaboration with specialized cardiac care centers is vital for patients with heart failure or cardiogenic shock. This collaboration ensures that the patient receives the most advanced and appropriate care, such as percutaneous coronary intervention (PCI), coronary artery bypass grafting (CABG), or heart transplant evaluation.

In summary, understanding the causes, clinical manifestations, and management strategies for heart failure and cardiogenic shock is essential for transport nurses and other healthcare professionals. Providing optimal care during transport, including pharmacological interventions, mechanical circulatory support devices, and collaboration with specialized cardiac care centers, can significantly improve patient outcomes in these critical situations.

Cardiac arrhythmias refer to abnormal heart rhythms that can range from benign to life-threatening. Managing arrhythmias during patient transport is crucial as they can impact hemodynamic stability and overall patient outcomes.

Types of Cardiac Arrhythmias: Arrhythmias can be classified based on their origin (atrial, junctional, or ventricular) and their rate (bradycardia or tachycardia). Some common arrhythmias include atrial fibrillation, atrial flutter, supraventricular tachycardia (SVT), ventricular tachycardia (VT), and ventricular fibrillation (VF).

Hemodynamic Impact: The impact of an arrhythmia on hemodynamic stability depends on its rate, regularity, and underlying cardiac function. Rapid or irregular rhythms can compromise cardiac output, leading to symptoms like dizziness, chest pain, shortness of breath, or even syncope. In severe cases, arrhythmias can result in hemodynamic instability, shock, or cardiac arrest.

Interventions for Arrhythmias: During patient transport, it's essential to identify and manage arrhythmias promptly. Interventions include electrical therapy and antiarrhythmic medications.

1. Electrical Therapy:
    - Defibrillation: This procedure delivers an electrical shock to the heart to treat life-threatening ventricular arrhythmias like VF and pulseless VT. Early defibrillation is crucial for improving survival rates in these patients.
    - Cardioversion: This technique uses synchronized electrical shocks to convert certain tachyarrhythmias (e.g., atrial fibrillation or flutter, and stable VT) back to a normal rhythm. It may be performed either electively or emergently, depending on the patient's clinical condition.
    - Pacing: Transcutaneous or transvenous pacing can be employed to manage bradyarrhythmias or unstable tachyarrhythmias with a slow ventricular response. Pacing helps maintain an adequate heart rate and, consequently, preserves cardiac output.
2. Antiarrhythmic Medications: Pharmacological agents can be used to manage various arrhythmias. Some examples include:
    - Adenosine for paroxysmal SVT.
    - Calcium channel blockers or beta-blockers for rate control in atrial fibrillation.

- Amiodarone or lidocaine for ventricular arrhythmias.

In summary, understanding the types of cardiac arrhythmias, their hemodynamic impact, and the appropriate interventions during patient transport is crucial for healthcare professionals. Timely management of arrhythmias using electrical therapy and antiarrhythmic medications can significantly improve patient outcomes and ensure safe transport.

Acute aortic syndromes are life-threatening vascular emergencies that involve the aorta, the body's main artery. They include aortic dissection and ruptured aortic aneurysm. Rapid diagnosis, stabilization, and transport to a specialized center for definitive care are essential for improving patient outcomes.

Pathophysiology:

- Aortic Dissection: This occurs when a tear forms in the inner layer of the aorta, allowing blood to enter and separate the layers, creating a false lumen. The dissection can propagate along the aorta, compromising blood flow to critical organs and potentially leading to rupture.
- Ruptured Aortic Aneurysm: An aneurysm is a localized dilation of the aortic wall. When the weakened wall ruptures, it results in massive hemorrhage and often proves fatal.

Clinical Presentation: Patients with acute aortic syndromes may exhibit various symptoms, some of which are common to both conditions:

- Sudden, severe chest or back pain, often described as tearing or ripping.
- Unequal blood pressures or pulses in the upper extremities.
- Altered mental status, syncope, or signs of shock.

Management Strategies:

1. Rapid Diagnosis: Time is of the essence in managing acute aortic syndromes. A high index of suspicion is necessary for prompt diagnosis. Diagnostic tools like point-of-care ultrasound or computed tomography (CT) scans can be helpful but may not be readily available during transport.
2. Stabilization: Initial management focuses on stabilizing the patient's hemodynamics and addressing any life-threatening complications:
   - Administer IV fluids cautiously to maintain adequate blood pressure without exacerbating bleeding or dissection.
   - Use vasodilators, such as nitroglycerin or sodium nitroprusside, to reduce blood pressure and shear forces on the aortic wall. Target a systolic blood pressure of 100-120 mmHg.
   - Administer pain relief to alleviate discomfort and reduce sympathetic stimulation.
   - Consider beta-blockers to reduce heart rate and blood pressure, provided there are no contraindications.
3. Transport to a Specialized Center: It is crucial to transport patients with acute aortic syndromes to a specialized center that can provide definitive care, including endovascular or open surgical repair, depending on the patient's condition and anatomy.

In conclusion, understanding the pathophysiology, clinical presentation, and management of acute aortic syndromes is vital for healthcare professionals. Rapid diagnosis, stabilization, and transport to a specialized center for definitive care are critical components in the management of these life-threatening conditions.

Chapter 4: Medical Emergencies

The Medical Emergencies chapter provides an overview of various non-traumatic medical conditions that may require emergency care and transportation. The chapter highlights the importance of rapid assessment, accurate diagnosis, and appropriate management of these conditions to improve patient outcomes. Key topics covered in this chapter include:

1. Respiratory Emergencies: This section addresses common respiratory issues such as asthma, chronic obstructive pulmonary disease (COPD), pneumonia, and pulmonary embolism. It emphasizes the importance of airway management, oxygen therapy, and pharmacological interventions.

2. Cardiovascular Emergencies: This section discusses acute coronary syndromes, heart failure, cardiogenic shock, cardiac arrhythmias, and acute aortic syndromes. It highlights the significance of early recognition, electrocardiogram (ECG) monitoring, pharmacological interventions, and coordination with specialized cardiac care centers.

3. Neurological Emergencies: This section focuses on conditions such as stroke, seizures, and altered mental status. It underscores the importance of rapid assessment, neurological examination, and timely transport to appropriate facilities for specialized care.

4. Endocrine Emergencies: This section covers emergencies related to endocrine system imbalances, such as diabetic ketoacidosis, hyperglycemic hyperosmolar state, and hypoglycemia. It highlights the significance of recognizing symptoms, monitoring blood glucose levels, and administering appropriate treatments.

5. Abdominal and Gastrointestinal Emergencies: This section discusses conditions such as gastrointestinal bleeding, acute abdomen, and bowel obstructions. It emphasizes the importance of prompt assessment, pain management, and transport to suitable healthcare facilities.

6. Toxicological Emergencies: This section covers poisoning and overdose situations, including drug, alcohol, and chemical exposures. It focuses on recognizing symptoms, providing supportive care, administering antidotes when applicable, and coordinating with poison control centers.

7. Environmental Emergencies: This section addresses emergencies caused by exposure to extreme temperatures, such as heat stroke, hypothermia, and frostbite. It highlights the importance of rapid recognition, appropriate cooling or warming measures, and fluid resuscitation when needed.

8. Infectious Diseases and Sepsis: This section discusses the presentation and management of severe infections and sepsis, emphasizing early recognition, administration of antibiotics, and aggressive fluid resuscitation.

Overall, the Medical Emergencies chapter aims to equip healthcare professionals with the knowledge and skills necessary to assess and manage a wide range of non-traumatic medical conditions effectively during emergency care and transportation.

Respiratory emergencies encompass a variety of conditions that can cause distress and life-threatening complications. To explore this topic thoroughly, let's delve into some common respiratory emergencies, their clinical presentations, and essential management steps.

1. Asthma Exacerbation: This occurs when airways become inflamed, narrowed, and filled with mucus, causing shortness of breath, wheezing, and chest tightness. Management includes administering inhaled bronchodilators (e.g., albuterol), supplemental oxygen, and corticosteroids. In severe cases, intravenous magnesium sulfate and continuous positive airway pressure (CPAP) might be necessary.

2. Chronic Obstructive Pulmonary Disease (COPD) Exacerbation: Characterized by increased shortness of breath, cough, and sputum production, COPD exacerbations can be triggered by infections or environmental factors. Management involves administering bronchodilators, corticosteroids, and supplemental oxygen. Non-invasive ventilation (NIV) may be required for patients with severe respiratory distress.

3. Pneumonia: Infection in the lungs can lead to symptoms such as fever, cough, shortness of breath, and chest pain. Management includes administering oxygen therapy, monitoring vital signs, and providing intravenous fluids and antibiotics as needed.

4. Pulmonary Embolism (PE): A blood clot in the lung's arteries can cause sudden shortness of breath, chest pain, and low blood oxygen levels. Management involves administering oxygen therapy, monitoring vital signs, providing intravenous fluids, and initiating anticoagulation therapy. In severe cases, thrombolytics or surgical intervention might be necessary.

5. Tension Pneumothorax: A buildup of air in the pleural space can cause lung collapse, leading to severe shortness of breath, chest pain, and hypotension. Management requires rapid needle decompression followed by chest tube insertion to relieve pressure and re-expand the lung.

In all respiratory emergencies, the primary goals are to ensure airway patency, optimize oxygenation and ventilation, and provide appropriate pharmacological interventions. Early recognition and prompt treatment are crucial in preventing complications and improving patient outcomes.

Acute coronary syndromes (ACS) encompass a spectrum of conditions resulting from insufficient blood supply to the heart muscle. To understand ACS more deeply, let's explore the pathophysiology, clinical manifestations, and prehospital management, emphasizing early recognition, ECG monitoring, and coordination with specialized cardiac care centers.
Pathophysiology: ACS typically occurs due to a rupture or erosion of atherosclerotic plaque in the coronary arteries, leading to blood clot formation and subsequent obstruction of blood flow. This can cause ischemia (insufficient oxygen supply) or infarction (death of heart muscle cells). ACS is classified into three categories: unstable angina (UA), non-ST elevation myocardial infarction (NSTEMI), and ST-elevation myocardial infarction (STEMI).
Clinical Manifestations: Common symptoms include chest pain or discomfort, radiating pain to the arms, neck, jaw, or back, shortness of breath, sweating, nausea, and lightheadedness. The nature and severity of symptoms may vary, and some individuals, particularly women, elderly, and diabetic patients, may present with atypical symptoms.

Prehospital Management: Early recognition and prompt intervention are critical in ACS. The following steps are essential for prehospital care:

1. Obtain a thorough patient history and perform a physical examination, assessing for signs of heart failure, shock, or other complications.
2. Administer oxygen therapy if the patient is hypoxic or in respiratory distress.
3. Perform a 12-lead ECG to detect ischemia or infarction, allowing for early diagnosis and appropriate treatment. Serial ECGs may be necessary to monitor changes.
4. Provide pharmacological interventions, such as aspirin, nitroglycerin, and possibly morphine or other analgesics for pain relief. In some cases, prehospital administration of antiplatelet and anticoagulant medications may be indicated.
5. Establish communication with a specialized cardiac care center for consultation and coordination, ensuring that the patient is transported to an appropriate facility for definitive care, including percutaneous coronary intervention (PCI) or fibrinolytic therapy, as necessary.

By understanding the complexities of ACS and implementing timely prehospital management strategies, healthcare providers can significantly impact patient outcomes, reducing morbidity and mortality associated with these life-threatening conditions.

Neurological emergencies, including stroke and seizures, demand rapid assessment and intervention by healthcare providers. Timely transportation to appropriate facilities for specialized care is crucial. Let's examine these neurological emergencies and the essential steps in their management.

Stroke: A stroke occurs when blood flow to a part of the brain is disrupted, leading to cell death and potentially permanent neurological deficits. There are two main types of stroke: ischemic (caused by a blocked blood vessel) and hemorrhagic (caused by a ruptured blood vessel).

Rapid Assessment: When a stroke is suspected, use the acronym FAST (Face, Arms, Speech, Time) to assess the patient:

Face: Ask the patient to smile and check for facial drooping.
Arms: Ask the patient to raise both arms and check for weakness or drifting.
Speech: Ask the patient to repeat a simple phrase and check for slurred or garbled speech.
Time: Note the time of symptom onset, as this is crucial for determining treatment eligibility.
Neurological Examination: Perform a more comprehensive neurological assessment, including evaluating the level of consciousness, motor and sensory function, coordination, and cranial nerves.

Transportation: Immediately transport the patient to a stroke center for specialized care. Time is of the essence, as treatments like thrombolytics (clot-busting drugs) have a narrow time window for administration.

Seizures: Seizures are caused by abnormal electrical activity in the brain and can be classified as focal (limited to one part of the brain) or generalized (involving both hemispheres). The most well-known type is the generalized tonic-clonic seizure, characterized by loss of consciousness, muscle rigidity, and convulsions.

Rapid Assessment: In the case of a seizure, ensure the patient's safety by moving them away from potential hazards and placing them in a recovery position. Assess airway, breathing, and circulation, and administer oxygen if needed.

Neurological Examination: Once the seizure has ended, perform a neurological assessment to determine the patient's level of consciousness, motor and sensory function, and cranial nerves. Also, assess for any underlying causes, such as hypoglycemia, fever, or head injury.

Transportation: Transport the patient to a healthcare facility for further evaluation and management, especially if it's the patient's first seizure, if there are recurring seizures, or if there are concerns about the underlying cause.

By understanding neurological emergencies and implementing prompt assessment and intervention strategies, healthcare providers can significantly impact patient outcomes and minimize potential complications.

Endocrine emergencies, such as diabetic ketoacidosis (DKA), hyperglycemic hyperosmolar state (HHS), and hypoglycemia, require prompt recognition and appropriate management. Let's delve into these conditions, their symptoms, and the necessary interventions.

1. Diabetic Ketoacidosis (DKA): DKA is a severe complication of diabetes, typically occurring in type 1 diabetes. It results from a combination of insulin deficiency and increased counter-regulatory hormones, leading to hyperglycemia, ketosis, and metabolic acidosis.

Symptoms: DKA presents with polyuria, polydipsia, nausea, vomiting, abdominal pain, rapid breathing (Kussmaul respirations), fruity-smelling breath, and altered mental status.

Management: Monitor blood glucose levels, vital signs, and electrolytes. Administer insulin and fluids to correct hyperglycemia, dehydration, and electrolyte imbalances. Ensure airway patency and administer oxygen if needed.

2. Hyperglycemic Hyperosmolar State (HHS): HHS, typically seen in type 2 diabetes, is characterized by severe hyperglycemia and dehydration without significant ketoacidosis.

Symptoms: HHS presents with polyuria, polydipsia, weakness, altered mental status, and dehydration. It can progress to seizures, coma, or even death if left untreated.

Management: Monitor blood glucose levels, vital signs, and electrolytes. Administer fluids to correct dehydration and insulin to lower blood glucose levels. Ensure airway patency and administer oxygen if needed.

3. Hypoglycemia: Hypoglycemia occurs when blood glucose levels fall below the normal range, often due to excessive insulin, missed meals, or increased physical activity.

Symptoms: Hypoglycemia presents with tremors, sweating, palpitations, confusion, irritability, dizziness, and even loss of consciousness.

Management: Check blood glucose levels to confirm hypoglycemia. For conscious patients, provide a source of sugar (e.g., fruit juice, candy, or glucose gel). For unconscious patients or those unable to swallow, administer intramuscular glucagon or intravenous dextrose. Recheck blood glucose levels and monitor vital signs.

Understanding endocrine emergencies and their appropriate management is crucial for healthcare providers. Proper recognition of symptoms, monitoring of blood glucose levels, and administration of suitable treatments can significantly impact patient outcomes and prevent life-threatening complications.

Toxicological and environmental emergencies encompass a wide range of situations, including poisoning, overdoses, and exposure to harmful substances or conditions. Let's discuss the essential principles for managing these emergencies, focusing on symptom recognition, supportive care, and administration of appropriate antidotes or interventions.

1. Poisoning: Poisoning occurs when a toxic substance is ingested, inhaled, or absorbed through the skin, causing harmful effects on the body.

Symptoms: The presentation of poisoning varies depending on the substance involved. Common symptoms include nausea, vomiting, abdominal pain, dizziness, altered mental status, seizures, and respiratory distress.

Management: Ensure scene safety and personal protective equipment usage. Assess and maintain airway, breathing, and circulation. Obtain a thorough history and identify the substance, if possible. Provide supportive care and follow specific antidote or intervention guidelines, if applicable. Transport to the appropriate healthcare facility.

2. Overdoses: Overdoses occur when an excessive amount of medication or drug is taken, causing potentially life-threatening effects.

Symptoms: Overdose symptoms vary based on the substance involved but may include drowsiness, confusion, agitation, seizures, respiratory depression, or cardiovascular instability.

Management: Assess and maintain airway, breathing, and circulation. Administer oxygen and provide ventilation support if necessary. Obtain a detailed history and attempt to identify the substance involved. Administer specific antidotes, if available and appropriate (e.g., naloxone for opioid overdose). Transport the patient to a suitable healthcare facility.

3. Environmental Emergencies: These emergencies arise from exposure to harmful environmental conditions, such as extreme temperatures, venomous bites, or hazardous materials.

Symptoms: Environmental emergencies can present with a wide array of symptoms depending on the exposure, including fever, chills, skin irritation, burns, difficulty breathing, or altered mental status.

Management: Ensure scene safety and personal protective equipment usage. Assess and maintain airway, breathing, and circulation. Remove the patient from the harmful environment or source of exposure, if possible. Administer supportive care, such as cooling measures for heat-related emergencies or warming measures for cold-related emergencies. Follow specific guidelines for the management of venomous bites or hazardous material exposures, if applicable. Transport the patient to the appropriate healthcare facility.

In summary, managing toxicological and environmental emergencies requires prompt recognition of symptoms, provision of supportive care, and administration of specific antidotes or interventions when appropriate. These steps are crucial in ensuring the best possible outcomes for patients in these challenging situations.

Chapter 5: Environmental and Trauma Emergencies

The Environmental and Trauma Emergencies chapter provides an in-depth understanding of various emergencies arising from environmental factors and physical injuries. It covers the assessment, management, and treatment of patients exposed to harmful environmental conditions or who have sustained traumatic injuries. The chapter is organized into several sections, focusing on the following topics:

1. Temperature-related emergencies: This section discusses heat-related emergencies, such as heat exhaustion and heatstroke, as well as cold-related emergencies, like hypothermia and frostbite. It emphasizes the importance of early recognition, intervention, and supportive care in these situations.
2. Drowning and near-drowning: This section covers the pathophysiology, assessment, and management of drowning and near-drowning incidents. It emphasizes the importance of rapid intervention, airway management, and resuscitation efforts.
3. Bites and stings: This section explores the management of various animal and insect bites and stings, including venomous and non-venomous encounters. It discusses the appropriate interventions and treatment, focusing on the recognition of symptoms, wound care, and administration of specific antidotes, if necessary.
4. High altitude emergencies: This section discusses the pathophysiology and management of altitude-related illnesses, such as acute mountain sickness, high-altitude cerebral edema, and high-altitude pulmonary edema. It emphasizes the importance of acclimatization, prevention, and appropriate treatment strategies.
5. Traumatic injuries: This section focuses on the assessment and management of various types of traumatic injuries, including blunt and penetrating trauma, head and spinal injuries, chest and abdominal trauma, and musculoskeletal injuries. It highlights the importance of rapid assessment, stabilization, and transportation to the appropriate healthcare facility for definitive care.

By understanding the various environmental and trauma emergencies, healthcare providers can be better prepared to assess, manage, and treat patients in these situations, ultimately improving patient outcomes.

Temperature-related emergencies can be quite challenging, but understanding the differences between heat exhaustion, heatstroke, hypothermia, and frostbite is crucial for providing proper care. So, let's dive into each condition and the best practices for their management.

Heat Exhaustion:
Heat exhaustion occurs when the body's temperature rises due to excessive heat exposure, resulting in symptoms like heavy sweating, dizziness, headache, and weakness. To manage heat exhaustion, move the person to a cooler environment and have them rest. Encourage them to drink cool, non-alcoholic fluids, and remove any tight or excess clothing. Applying cool, wet towels to the skin can also help.

Heatstroke:

Heatstroke is a more severe form of heat exhaustion and can be life-threatening. It occurs when the body's temperature rises above 104°F (40°C) and presents symptoms such as hot, dry skin, rapid pulse, and confusion. In case of heatstroke, call for emergency medical assistance immediately. Meanwhile, initiate rapid cooling by spraying the person with water, applying ice packs to the neck, armpits, and groin, and fanning the person to promote heat loss through evaporation.

Hypothermia:

Hypothermia occurs when the body's temperature drops below 95°F (35°C) due to cold exposure. Signs of hypothermia include shivering, confusion, and slowed breathing. To manage hypothermia, remove the person from the cold environment and remove any wet clothing. Wrap the person in blankets, and provide warm, non-alcoholic fluids if they are conscious. Do not apply direct heat, like heating pads or hot water, as this may cause tissue damage.

Frostbite:

Frostbite happens when the skin and underlying tissues freeze due to extreme cold. It typically affects extremities like fingers, toes, nose, and ears. Symptoms include numbness, pale or blue-gray skin, and hard, cold skin. To manage frostbite, gently rewarm the affected area using warm water (not hot) or body heat, such as placing frostbitten fingers in the armpit. Do not rub or massage the affected area, as this may cause further tissue damage. Seek medical attention promptly.

When dealing with temperature-related emergencies, always remember to protect yourself from the extreme conditions as well. Additionally, prevention is key: wearing appropriate clothing, staying hydrated, and avoiding excessive exposure to extreme temperatures can reduce the risk of these emergencies occurring in the first place.

Drowning and near-drowning incidents are critical emergencies that require immediate intervention. Let's delve into the pathophysiology, assessment, and management of these situations, as well as the potential complications and long-term outcomes.

Pathophysiology:

Drowning occurs when a person's airway is submerged in a liquid, typically water, leading to asphyxia and the inability to breathe. In near-drowning situations, a person may still be alive but at risk for severe complications. When a person is submerged, they may experience laryngospasm, a reflexive closure of the vocal cords, which can initially prevent water from entering the lungs. However, if the laryngospasm relaxes or is overcome by the water pressure, water will enter the lungs, impairing gas exchange and causing hypoxia, which can lead to organ damage and death.

Assessment:

When you encounter a drowning or near-drowning victim, first ensure scene safety and do not enter the water if it puts you at risk. Quickly assess the person's responsiveness, breathing, and circulation. If the victim is unresponsive or not breathing, initiate resuscitation efforts immediately.

Management:
In drowning or near-drowning situations, time is of the essence. Rapid intervention is crucial. If the victim is not breathing, begin CPR with a focus on providing rescue breaths. This is because drowning victims typically suffer from a lack of oxygen rather than circulatory failure. Once the victim is removed from the water, continue CPR and use an automated external defibrillator (AED) if available and indicated.

Potential Complications:
Complications from drowning and near-drowning incidents can be severe and may include acute respiratory distress syndrome (ARDS), aspiration pneumonia, and electrolyte imbalances. Hypoxic brain injury is another significant concern, which may result in long-term neurological deficits or death.

Long-term Outcomes:
The long-term outcomes for drowning and near-drowning victims depend on several factors, including the duration of submersion, water temperature, and the quality of immediate resuscitation efforts. Cold water submersion may offer some protection, as it slows metabolic processes and can prolong the window for successful resuscitation. However, even with prompt and proper care, some victims may experience lasting neurological damage or other long-term health issues.

In summary, understanding drowning and near-drowning incidents is crucial for providing rapid and effective care. Early intervention, proper airway management, and resuscitation efforts can significantly impact the patient's outcome and long-term quality of life.

Bites and stings from animals and insects can range from minor irritations to life-threatening emergencies. Let's examine various types of bites and stings, their treatments, and the role of healthcare providers in managing these emergencies.
Venomous Bites and Stings: Venomous creatures, such as snakes, spiders, and some insects, can inject venom through their bites or stings, which may lead to severe local and systemic reactions. Treatment depends on the specific species involved and the severity of the reaction.
1. Snakebites: Not all snakebites involve venom injection, but it is crucial to assume that venom is present. Keep the victim calm and immobile, and seek immediate medical attention. Do not apply a tourniquet or attempt to suck out the venom, as these actions may worsen the situation.
2. Spider bites: Bites from venomous spiders, like black widows or brown recluses, can cause significant local tissue damage and systemic symptoms. Clean the bite area with soap and water, apply a cold compress, and elevate the affected limb. Seek medical attention for severe reactions or if the victim is a child, elderly, or has underlying health issues.

3. Insect stings: Stings from bees, wasps, or hornets can cause pain, swelling, and, in some cases, anaphylactic reactions. Remove the stinger if present, wash the area, and apply a cold pack. Over-the-counter pain relievers and antihistamines can help with mild to moderate symptoms. For severe reactions, such as difficulty breathing, call 911 and administer an epinephrine autoinjector if available.

Non-Venomous Bites and Stings: Non-venomous bites, like those from dogs, cats, or other animals, can still cause injury and infection. Clean the wound with soap and water, apply an antibiotic ointment, and cover it with a sterile bandage. Seek medical attention for deep wounds, punctures, or if signs of infection develop.

The Role of Healthcare Providers: In managing bite and sting emergencies, healthcare providers play a critical role in assessing the severity of the injury, administering appropriate treatments, and monitoring the patient for complications. In some cases, providers may administer antivenom or other medications, such as antibiotics or tetanus prophylaxis.

In conclusion, understanding various bites and stings, their potential complications, and appropriate treatment strategies is essential for providing effective care. Healthcare providers play a crucial role in managing these emergencies and preventing further harm.

High-altitude emergencies are challenging situations that can develop when individuals ascend to significant elevations. Let's delve into the pathophysiology, prevention, and management of altitude-related illnesses, along with acclimatization strategies and the importance of early symptom recognition.

Pathophysiology: The primary cause of altitude-related illnesses is the reduced atmospheric pressure and lower oxygen levels at high altitudes. The body attempts to adapt to these conditions through various physiological changes. However, if the ascent is too rapid, these adaptations may be insufficient, leading to acute mountain sickness (AMS), high-altitude cerebral edema (HACE), or high-altitude pulmonary edema (HAPE).

1. Acute Mountain Sickness (AMS): AMS is a common condition characterized by symptoms like headache, nausea, dizziness, and fatigue. It usually occurs above 8,000 feet (2,500 meters) and is caused by inadequate acclimatization.
2. High-Altitude Cerebral Edema (HACE): HACE is a severe form of AMS and occurs when fluid accumulates in the brain, causing confusion, ataxia, and altered consciousness. It is a life-threatening condition requiring immediate descent and medical intervention.
3. High-Altitude Pulmonary Edema (HAPE): HAPE is caused by fluid build-up in the lungs due to increased pressure in the pulmonary blood vessels. Symptoms include shortness of breath, cough, chest pain, and fatigue. Like HACE, HAPE is a potentially fatal condition that necessitates urgent descent and medical care.

Prevention and Acclimatization: The best strategy for preventing altitude-related illnesses is gradual acclimatization, allowing the body to adjust to the lower oxygen levels. Recommendations include:

1. Slow ascent: Increase elevation gradually, ideally no more than 1,000 feet (300 meters) per day above 8,000 feet (2,500 meters).
2. "Climb high, sleep low": Climb to a higher altitude during the day but sleep at a lower elevation to promote acclimatization.
3. Stay hydrated: Drink plenty of water to maintain proper hydration.

4. Medications: In some cases, healthcare providers may recommend prophylactic medications like acetazolamide to help with acclimatization.

Management: Recognizing symptoms early and taking appropriate action is critical for managing altitude-related illnesses. Key steps include:

1. Descent: If symptoms of AMS, HACE, or HAPE develop, descend to a lower altitude immediately. This is often the most effective treatment.
2. Oxygen: Supplemental oxygen can help alleviate symptoms and improve oxygen saturation.
3. Medications: Healthcare providers may administer medications like dexamethasone for HACE or nifedipine for HAPE to alleviate symptoms and stabilize the patient during descent.

In summary, understanding the pathophysiology, prevention, and management of altitude-related illnesses is essential for staying safe in high-altitude environments. Acclimatization strategies and early symptom recognition are crucial for minimizing risks and ensuring appropriate care when emergencies arise.

Traumatic injuries can encompass a wide range of situations and can vary in severity. To effectively manage these emergencies, it's essential to understand the assessment and management of different types of injuries, including blunt and penetrating trauma, head and spinal injuries, chest and abdominal trauma, and musculoskeletal injuries. Let's explore each of these categories and discuss rapid assessment, stabilization, and transportation to appropriate healthcare facilities.

1. Blunt and penetrating trauma: Blunt trauma results from a forceful impact that doesn't break the skin, while penetrating trauma occurs when an object pierces the skin and enters the body. Both types require rapid assessment to identify life-threatening injuries. In cases of blunt trauma, look for signs of internal bleeding, fractures, or organ damage. For penetrating trauma, control external bleeding and assess for damage to internal organs or major blood vessels.
2. Head and spinal injuries: Traumatic brain injuries (TBIs) can range from mild concussions to severe life-threatening injuries. Assess the level of consciousness using the AVPU (Alert, Verbal, Painful, Unresponsive) scale or Glasgow Coma Scale (GCS). Stabilize the patient's head and neck to prevent further spinal damage. For spinal injuries, maintain spinal immobilization using a cervical collar or other stabilization devices.
3. Chest and abdominal trauma: Injuries to the chest and abdomen can be life-threatening, as they may involve vital organs and major blood vessels. Assess for signs of pneumothorax, hemothorax, or internal bleeding. In cases of tension pneumothorax, needle decompression may be necessary. Rapidly assess the abdomen for rigidity, distension, or bruising, which may indicate internal injury.
4. Musculoskeletal injuries: These injuries include fractures, dislocations, and sprains. Assess for deformity, swelling, and discoloration. Immobilize the injured area with splints or bandages, apply ice to reduce swelling, and elevate the injured limb if possible. Pain management may be necessary, depending on the severity of the injury.

In all cases, the primary focus should be on rapid assessment and stabilization. Follow the ABCDE approach: Airway, Breathing, Circulation, Disability, and Exposure. Ensure the patient's airway is clear and unobstructed, evaluate their breathing and circulation, assess for neurological deficits, and expose any injuries to facilitate examination.

Once the initial assessment and stabilization are complete, arrange for transportation to an appropriate healthcare facility for definitive care. This may involve coordinating with emergency medical services (EMS) or specialized trauma centers.

In summary, managing traumatic injuries requires a comprehensive understanding of different types of injuries and the appropriate assessment, stabilization, and management strategies. Rapid intervention and coordination with healthcare facilities are essential for optimizing patient outcomes.

Burn injuries can result from various sources, such as heat, chemicals, electricity, and radiation. They vary in severity and can have serious consequences if not managed properly. To effectively treat burn injuries, it's crucial to understand the classification of burns, the initial assessment, and the appropriate management techniques.

Classification of burns:

Burns are classified according to their depth, as follows:

a. First-degree burns: These affect the outer layer of the skin (epidermis) and cause redness, mild swelling, and pain. Sunburn is a common example of a first-degree burn.

b. Second-degree burns: These burns extend through the epidermis and into the dermis (the second layer of skin), causing blisters, swelling, and severe pain. They are further divided into superficial and deep second-degree burns, depending on the extent of dermal involvement.

c. Third-degree burns: These are full-thickness burns that destroy both the epidermis and dermis, reaching the underlying tissues. They appear white, brown, or black and may have a leathery texture. Pain may be absent due to nerve damage.

d. Fourth-degree burns: These are the most severe and extend beyond the skin, affecting muscles, tendons, and even bones. They are typically black and charred, with no sensation in the affected area.

Initial assessment:

When assessing a burn injury, follow the ABCDE approach (Airway, Breathing, Circulation, Disability, Exposure) to ensure the patient's vital functions are stable. Assess the extent of the burn by estimating the total body surface area (TBSA) affected, using the "rule of nines" or the palm method. Also, evaluate the depth and source of the burn, as this will guide management.

Burn management:

The appropriate management of burn injuries depends on the severity and type of burn. Here are some general guidelines:

a. First-degree burns: Cool the burn with cold running water for at least 10-20 minutes, then apply a moisturizing lotion or aloe vera to soothe the skin. Avoid using ice, as it can cause further damage. Over-the-counter pain relievers may help alleviate discomfort.

b. Second-degree burns: Cool the burn as for first-degree burns, but avoid breaking any blisters, as this increases the risk of infection. Apply a sterile, non-adherent dressing to protect the wound, and elevate the affected area if possible. Pain management and tetanus prophylaxis may be necessary.

c. Third- and fourth-degree burns: Do not apply water or ointments to these burns, as they require specialized care. Cover the burn with a clean, dry, non-adherent dressing or cloth, and seek immediate medical attention. Elevate the affected area and provide pain management as needed.

d. Chemical burns: Remove any contaminated clothing and brush off any dry chemicals. Flush the affected area with copious amounts of water for at least 20 minutes, ensuring the water does not come into contact with unaffected skin. Seek medical attention promptly.

e. Electrical burns: Turn off the power source and ensure the scene is safe before approaching the patient. Electrical burns may cause internal injuries that are not immediately visible, so seek medical attention immediately.

In all cases, monitor the patient for signs of shock and address any other injuries. Seek professional medical help for severe burns, chemical burns, or electrical burns, as they often require specialized care.

In summary, the effective management of burn injuries involves understanding the classification of burns, conducting a thorough assessment, and applying appropriate treatment techniques. Always seek medical help for severe or specialized burns to ensure optimal patient outcomes.

Chapter 6: Special Populations

The Special Populations chapter focuses on the unique considerations, challenges, and approaches needed when providing emergency care to specific groups of individuals. These populations may have different physiological, psychological, or social needs that require tailored assessment and management techniques. Key topics covered in this chapter include:

1. Pediatric Emergencies: This section discusses the anatomical and physiological differences between children and adults, which impact their response to illness and injury. It covers various pediatric emergencies, including respiratory distress, shock, and trauma, highlighting the importance of age-appropriate assessment and interventions.
2. Geriatric Emergencies: This section explores the unique challenges of managing emergencies in older adults. It emphasizes the importance of considering age-related changes, comorbidities, and medication use when assessing and treating geriatric patients. Topics include falls, delirium, and polypharmacy.
3. Obstetric and Gynecological Emergencies: This section delves into emergencies related to pregnancy and the female reproductive system. It discusses the assessment and management of conditions such as pre-eclampsia, eclampsia, and postpartum hemorrhage, as well as the provision of emergency childbirth assistance.
4. Mental Health Emergencies: This section covers the assessment and management of patients experiencing acute mental health crises, such as suicidal ideation, aggressive behavior, or psychosis. It emphasizes the importance of effective communication, de-escalation techniques, and collaboration with mental health professionals.
5. Patients with Disabilities: This section highlights the importance of understanding and accommodating the needs of patients with physical, cognitive, or sensory disabilities when providing emergency care. It discusses effective communication strategies and the importance of considering the patient's unique needs during assessment and treatment.
6. Cultural Competence and Sensitivity: This section focuses on the significance of cultural competence and sensitivity when providing care to diverse populations. It discusses communication strategies, cultural awareness, and the importance of respecting patients' beliefs and values during treatment.

By understanding the unique needs and challenges associated with these special populations, emergency care providers can tailor their assessment and management approaches to optimize patient outcomes and ensure respectful, patient-centered care.

Developing age-appropriate approaches when managing emergencies is crucial, as the unique needs of pediatric and geriatric patients greatly impact their response to illness and injury. Let's dive into effective assessment and management techniques for both age groups.
Pediatric Emergencies:

1. Airway Management: Children have smaller airways, making them more prone to obstruction. Use appropriately sized equipment, and be mindful of the head-tilt chin-lift technique, which may require a modified approach in infants.
2. Breathing Assessment: Children have faster respiratory rates and are more reliant on diaphragmatic breathing. Be prepared to provide respiratory support early.

3. Circulation: Children have higher heart rates and may compensate for shock longer than adults. Monitor for signs of decompensation and administer fluids or medications accordingly.
4. Developmental Considerations: Assess pain and discomfort using age-appropriate pain scales, and communicate with the child at their developmental level. Involve parents or caregivers when possible.
5. Emotional Support: Create a calming environment, use simple language, and provide comfort items when appropriate.

Geriatric Emergencies:
1. Airway Management: Be aware of dentures and potential difficulty in airway management due to anatomical changes associated with aging.
2. Breathing Assessment: Older patients may have reduced respiratory reserve, making it crucial to closely monitor their breathing and provide timely support.
3. Circulation: Age-related changes in blood vessels and cardiac function may affect the presentation of shock or other circulatory issues. Monitor vital signs closely and adjust interventions as needed.
4. Cognitive Impairments: Be prepared to encounter dementia, delirium, or other cognitive impairments. Use clear, simple language and reorient the patient as necessary.
5. Polypharmacy: Older patients often take multiple medications, which can increase the risk of drug interactions or adverse effects. Obtain a thorough medication history and consider potential drug-related issues during assessment and management.

By understanding the unique physiological and psychological aspects of pediatric and geriatric patients, healthcare providers can more effectively assess and manage emergencies in these age groups, ultimately improving patient outcomes.

Navigating obstetric and gynecological emergencies requires knowledge of the female reproductive system, pregnancy, and potential complications. Let's explore critical components of managing these emergencies.
1. Recognizing Signs and Symptoms: Be aware of common conditions and their manifestations, such as ectopic pregnancy (sharp abdominal pain, shoulder pain), spontaneous abortion (vaginal bleeding, cramping), and preeclampsia (hypertension, headache, blurred vision). Early identification can help guide appropriate interventions.
2. Emergency Childbirth Assistance: a. Preparing the Environment: Ensure privacy, warmth, and cleanliness. Assemble necessary supplies, like gloves, sterile towels, and suction devices. b. Assessing the Stage of Labor: Determine labor progress by assessing contraction frequency and duration, as well as cervical dilation. c. Delivery: Encourage the mother to push during contractions. Support the baby's head as it emerges, and clear the airway with suction. Guide the shoulders out, followed by the rest of the body. d. Post-Delivery Care: Clamp and cut the umbilical cord, assess and stimulate the baby, and ensure proper breathing. Keep the baby warm and initiate skin-to-skin contact with the mother. Monitor for the delivery of the placenta and manage postpartum bleeding.
3. Managing Complications: a. Breech Presentation: Seek immediate medical assistance if the baby's buttocks or feet appear first. Attempting a breech delivery in a prehospital setting is not recommended. b. Cord Prolapse: If the umbilical cord emerges before the

baby, instruct the mother to stop pushing and assume a knee-chest or head-down position. Seek immediate medical help. c. Postpartum Hemorrhage: Administer uterine massage and medications as prescribed to control bleeding, monitor vital signs, and transport the patient to the hospital for further evaluation.

4. Special Considerations: a. Multiple Births: Be prepared for the delivery of additional babies, and manage each birth individually. b. Preterm Labor: If a premature birth is imminent, provide support and promptly transport the mother and newborn(s) to a medical facility equipped to handle preterm deliveries.

By understanding the essentials of managing obstetric and gynecological emergencies, healthcare providers can better recognize and address complications, provide appropriate care, and help ensure the safety of both the mother and the baby.

Managing patients **experiencing acute mental health crises** is a vital skill for healthcare providers. Let's delve into the essential principles of assessment and management in these situations.

1. Effective Communication: Establishing rapport and trust is crucial. Approach the patient calmly, maintain a non-threatening body language, and use active listening. Validate the patient's feelings and show empathy, while avoiding judgment or confrontation.

2. Assessment: Perform a thorough assessment, including the patient's mental status, medical history, and potential risk factors for self-harm or harm to others. Identify any possible triggers or stressors, and consider any underlying medical conditions that may contribute to the crisis.

3. De-Escalation Techniques: a. Establish Boundaries: Maintain a safe distance, respect personal space, and avoid physical contact unless necessary. b. Be Patient: Give the person time to express themselves, and avoid interrupting or rushing the conversation. c. Offer Choices: Empower the patient by providing options when possible, reinforcing their sense of control and autonomy. d. Stay Calm: Remain composed, even if the patient becomes agitated or hostile. Your demeanor can influence their behavior.

4. Collaboration with Mental Health Professionals: Depending on the severity of the crisis, it may be necessary to involve mental health professionals, such as psychiatrists or crisis intervention teams. They can provide specialized assessment and care, as well as resources and support for the patient.

5. Safety Considerations: Always prioritize the safety of the patient, yourself, and others. If the situation escalates, and there is imminent risk, you may need to call for additional assistance, such as law enforcement or emergency medical services.

6. Documentation and Follow-Up: Accurately document the patient's mental health status, interventions provided, and any referrals made. Encourage the patient to seek follow-up care with mental health professionals and provide resources for support.

By understanding the essential principles of managing acute mental health crises, healthcare providers can better assess patients, employ de-escalation techniques, and collaborate with mental health professionals to ensure effective care and support.

Adapting emergency care to meet the needs of patients with disabilities is crucial for providing equitable healthcare. Here, we'll discuss key considerations and strategies for addressing physical, cognitive, or sensory disabilities in an emergency context.

1. Communication: a. Be Patient: Allow extra time for patients to communicate and express themselves. b. Use Simple Language: Speak clearly and use simple terms to ensure comprehension. c. Augmentative Communication: Utilize alternative communication methods, such as visual aids, gestures, or communication devices, to support understanding. d. Verify Comprehension: Confirm that the patient has understood your instructions or questions.

2. Accessibility: a. Physical Access: Ensure that your treatment space is accessible to patients with mobility impairments. This may include using ramps, wide doorways, or adjustable-height equipment. b. Sensory Adaptations: For patients with sensory disabilities, minimize distracting stimuli, such as loud noises or bright lights. Provide written materials in large print or Braille, and consider using hearing loops for those with hearing impairments.

3. Tailored Assessment and Treatment Approaches: a. Modify Techniques: Adapt your physical examination techniques to accommodate the patient's disability. For example, if a patient has limited mobility, consider alternative ways to assess vital signs or perform other assessments. b. Involve the Patient: Engage the patient in their care by asking about their preferences and accommodating their needs whenever possible. c. Coordinate Care: Collaborate with the patient's primary care providers or specialists to ensure continuity of care and a comprehensive understanding of their medical needs.

4. Cultural Competency and Sensitivity: a. Respect Autonomy: Acknowledge and respect the patient's independence and ability to make decisions about their care. b. Avoid Stereotyping: Do not make assumptions about a patient's abilities or needs based on their disability. Each patient is unique, and their experiences will differ. c. Educate Yourself: Familiarize yourself with various disabilities and the best practices for providing care to individuals with these disabilities.

By focusing on communication, accessibility, and tailored assessment and treatment approaches, healthcare providers can adapt emergency care to better serve patients with disabilities, ensuring that they receive equitable and effective care.

Cultural competence is a crucial skill for healthcare providers in emergency care settings, as it ensures effective communication and fosters a patient-centered approach. Here, we will delve into the importance of cultural competence and sensitivity, and explore the key aspects that contribute to its development.

1. Understanding Cultural Competence: a. Definition: Cultural competence refers to the ability to provide effective healthcare services to individuals from diverse backgrounds, taking into account their cultural beliefs, practices, and values. b. Importance: Cultural competence ensures that healthcare providers can work with diverse populations, avoid miscommunication, and promote patient satisfaction and trust.

2. Effective Communication Strategies: a. Active Listening: Pay close attention to the patient's concerns, and show empathy and understanding. b. Nonverbal Communication: Be aware of the potential cultural implications of body language, eye

contact, and personal space. c. Language Barriers: Utilize interpreter services, translation tools, or multilingual staff when necessary to facilitate communication.

3. Developing Cultural Awareness: a. Self-Assessment: Reflect on your own cultural biases and beliefs to better understand how they may impact patient care. b. Cultural Knowledge: Learn about different cultural practices, beliefs, and values to better anticipate and respect the needs of diverse patients. c. Open-Mindedness: Approach each patient with an open mind, and be receptive to learning about their unique cultural perspectives.

4. Respecting Patients' Beliefs and Values: a. Informed Consent: Ensure that patients understand their treatment options and are given the opportunity to make decisions based on their cultural beliefs and values. b. Spiritual and Cultural Practices: Accommodate patients' spiritual and cultural practices whenever possible, such as providing access to prayer spaces or accommodating dietary restrictions. c. Collaborative Decision-Making: Engage patients and their families in the decision-making process, and respect their preferences and choices.

Cultivating cultural competence in emergency care involves developing effective communication strategies, enhancing cultural awareness, and respecting patients' beliefs and values during treatment. By doing so, healthcare providers can create a more inclusive and patient-centered environment, leading to improved patient satisfaction and better health outcomes.

Chapter 7: Operations

The Operations chapter focuses on the practical aspects of emergency medical services (EMS), covering the essential components that ensure the efficient and safe delivery of care to patients. This overview will highlight key topics within the chapter, including:

1. EMS System Structure: This section describes the organization and components of an EMS system, including the roles and responsibilities of various personnel, communication networks, medical oversight, and public health integration.
2. Dispatch and Communication: This topic covers the vital role of emergency medical dispatchers, call prioritization, and effective communication between EMS providers, dispatch centers, and receiving facilities.
3. Scene Safety and Management: This section highlights the importance of maintaining scene safety, managing potential hazards, and coordinating with other responding agencies. Key aspects of scene management include personal protective equipment (PPE), hazard recognition, and proper resource utilization.
4. Patient Extrication and Transportation: This part of the chapter delves into patient extrication techniques, safe lifting and moving procedures, and the considerations for selecting appropriate transportation methods.
5. Triage and Mass Casualty Incidents (MCIs): This section discusses the principles of triage, strategies for managing MCIs, and the coordination with other agencies during large-scale emergencies.
6. Hazardous Materials (HazMat) and Decontamination: This topic covers the basics of hazardous materials, recognizing potential HazMat situations, and the importance of decontamination procedures for both patients and responders.
7. Incident Command System (ICS): This section introduces the ICS, its structure and principles, and the roles and responsibilities of EMS providers within the ICS during an emergency response.
8. Legal and Ethical Considerations: This part of the chapter explores the legal and ethical aspects of EMS operations, including patient consent, refusal of care, confidentiality, and documentation.

The Operations chapter is designed to provide a comprehensive understanding of the practical components of emergency medical services, ensuring EMS providers are well-equipped to deliver efficient and safe patient care in various situations.

An EMS system is a complex network of professionals working together to provide emergency care to patients in need. In order to ensure successful patient care, understanding the roles and responsibilities of each team member is crucial. Let's delve deeper into the various personnel involved, their specific duties, and the significance of collaboration and communication among them.

1. Emergency Medical Dispatchers (EMDs): EMDs are the first point of contact in an emergency situation. They receive emergency calls, gather vital information, prioritize calls based on severity, and dispatch appropriate EMS resources. EMDs also provide pre-

arrival instructions and support to callers, guiding them through life-saving interventions while awaiting EMS arrival.

2. Emergency Medical Responders (EMRs): EMRs are trained to provide basic, immediate care at the scene of an emergency. Their responsibilities include scene safety, initial patient assessment, and stabilization through interventions like CPR, bleeding control, and oxygen administration. EMRs work closely with higher-level EMS personnel and may assist in transferring patients to the ambulance.

3. Emergency Medical Technicians (EMTs): EMTs possess more advanced skills than EMRs and are capable of providing basic life support (BLS). They perform patient assessments, administer certain medications, and manage airway, breathing, and circulation issues. EMTs work closely with other EMS providers and transport patients to appropriate medical facilities.

4. Advanced Emergency Medical Technicians (AEMTs): AEMTs have a higher level of training than EMTs and can provide limited advanced life support (ALS) interventions. They're able to perform advanced airway management, administer additional medications, and initiate intravenous therapy, among other skills.

5. Paramedics: As the highest level of prehospital EMS providers, paramedics have the most extensive scope of practice. They can perform advanced assessments, administer a wider range of medications, and carry out invasive procedures. Paramedics coordinate with other healthcare professionals and determine the most suitable destination for patients, considering their specific medical needs.

6. EMS Supervisors and Medical Directors: These professionals oversee the EMS system, ensuring quality care, adherence to protocols, and continuous improvement. EMS supervisors manage field operations and personnel, while medical directors are responsible for developing protocols and providing medical oversight.

Collaboration and communication are essential for EMS personnel to work efficiently and effectively. Clear, concise communication ensures that necessary information is shared among team members, enabling them to make informed decisions and provide optimal patient care. Effective collaboration also fosters a supportive work environment and promotes a culture of continuous learning and improvement.

Effective communication is a cornerstone of successful emergency medical services (EMS), with emergency medical dispatchers (EMDs) playing a pivotal role. In this discussion, we'll delve into the vital role of EMDs, the process of call prioritization, and best practices for maintaining clear and concise communication between EMS providers, dispatch centers, and receiving facilities.

1. The Vital Role of Emergency Medical Dispatchers: EMDs serve as the initial point of contact for emergency calls. They gather essential information from callers, such as the nature of the emergency, location, and patient's condition. EMDs also provide pre-arrival instructions to callers, guiding them in performing life-saving interventions, like CPR, until EMS providers arrive on scene. They are responsible for coordinating the appropriate response and facilitating effective communication among all parties involved.

2. Call Prioritization: One of the key responsibilities of EMDs is to prioritize emergency calls based on their severity. They use a system called Emergency Medical Dispatch (EMD) to

categorize calls into different levels of urgency. This process helps ensure that the most critical cases receive prompt attention and resources are allocated efficiently. Call prioritization requires skillful judgment and decision-making, as well as familiarity with local EMS resources.

3. Best Practices for Clear and Concise Communication: a. Use Standardized Terminology: To avoid misunderstandings, EMS personnel should use standardized language and medical terminology. This helps ensure that all parties understand the information being communicated, even when working with personnel from different agencies or backgrounds.

b. Speak Clearly and Slowly: When conveying information, it's important to speak clearly and at a moderate pace. This allows everyone involved to process the information accurately and ask for clarification if needed.

c. Be Specific and Concise: To facilitate efficient communication, provide specific, concise details when describing a patient's condition, location, or other relevant information. Avoid using jargon, slang, or ambiguous terms.

d. Confirm Understanding: After relaying information, confirm that the message was understood by the recipient. This can be done by asking them to repeat back the information or by seeking verbal confirmation.

e. Utilize Closed-Loop Communication: This technique involves the sender of a message waiting for the recipient to acknowledge receipt and confirm understanding before considering the message complete. This process helps to minimize miscommunications and ensure that critical information is accurately conveyed.

By understanding the critical role of EMDs, the process of call prioritization, and best practices for clear communication, EMS providers can work together effectively, ensuring timely and efficient patient care.

Triage and management of mass casualty incidents (MCIs) require a systematic approach to ensure the most effective use of resources and timely care for patients. In this discussion, we will examine the concepts of triage, various triage systems, and strategies for effectively managing MCIs, including resource allocation and coordination with other responding agencies.

Triage: Triage is the process of rapidly assessing and prioritizing patients according to the severity of their injuries or medical conditions. The goal is to allocate limited resources in a way that maximizes the number of lives saved. Triage is essential during MCIs, where the number of patients often exceeds the available resources.

Triage Systems: Various triage systems have been developed to facilitate a consistent and efficient approach to patient assessment and prioritization. Some of the most commonly used systems include:

a. Simple Triage and Rapid Treatment (START): This system is designed for adult patients and involves assessing patients' ability to walk, their respiratory rate, and their mental status. Patients are then categorized into one of four color-coded priority levels: green (minor), yellow (delayed), red (immediate), or black (deceased or expectant).

b. JumpSTART Pediatric Triage: This system is an adaptation of START for pediatric patients. It includes age-specific modifications to account for differences in normal vital signs and physiological responses in children.

c. SALT (Sort, Assess, Lifesaving Interventions, Treatment/Transport) Triage: This system uses a similar approach to START and JumpSTART but adds an additional step to identify patients requiring immediate lifesaving interventions.

Strategies for Managing Mass Casualty Incidents:

a. Incident Command System (ICS): The ICS is a standardized approach to the command, control, and coordination of emergency response. It provides a structure for organizing and managing resources, establishing clear lines of communication, and defining roles and responsibilities.

b. Resource Allocation: During an MCI, it's crucial to allocate resources effectively to ensure the greatest benefit for the largest number of patients. This may involve prioritizing treatment and transport of the most critically injured patients or identifying and reallocating resources from other areas.

c. Coordination with Other Responding Agencies: Effective MCI management requires collaboration and communication with other responding agencies, such as law enforcement, fire departments, hospitals, and public health agencies. Establishing a unified command structure and maintaining open lines of communication can help ensure a coordinated response.

Legal and ethical considerations are crucial in EMS operations to ensure the protection of patients' rights and the adherence of EMS professionals to the highest standards of care. Let's delve into some key aspects:

1. Informed Consent: Before initiating treatment, it is important to obtain the patient's informed consent. This involves explaining the proposed treatment, its risks and benefits, and any available alternatives. For informed consent to be valid, the patient must have decision-making capacity, receive adequate information, and consent voluntarily.

2. Refusal of Care: Patients have the right to refuse care, even if it is against medical advice. EMS providers must respect this decision and inform the patient of potential consequences. In cases where the patient lacks decision-making capacity, providers must act in the best interest of the patient.

3. Patient Confidentiality: EMS providers are bound by the principles of patient confidentiality and must protect patient information from unauthorized disclosure. This includes maintaining the privacy of medical records, adhering to the Health Insurance Portability and Accountability Act (HIPAA) regulations, and only sharing patient information with authorized individuals for the purpose of continuity of care.

4. Accurate and Thorough Documentation: Accurate and complete documentation is essential in EMS for several reasons, such as ensuring continuity of care, supporting billing and reimbursement, and providing legal protection for EMS providers. Documentation should include a thorough patient assessment, interventions performed, response to treatment, and any relevant communication with other healthcare providers.

5. Other legal and ethical considerations: EMS providers should also be familiar with mandatory reporting requirements, issues related to end-of-life care, and relevant local and federal laws governing their practice. Understanding these principles and applying them in clinical practice is essential for delivering high-quality care while minimizing the risk of legal complications.

Chapter 8: Test Preparation and Study Tips

Preparing for the CFRN exam can be challenging, but with the right approach and study habits, you can increase your chances of success. Here are some study tips and test-taking strategies to help you prepare:

Study Tips:

1. Understand the exam format: Familiarize yourself with the CFRN exam structure and the topics covered. Knowing what to expect will help you allocate your study time efficiently.
2. Create a study schedule: Plan your study time in advance and stick to a consistent schedule. Break the material into manageable sections and allocate enough time for each topic.
3. Use multiple resources: Utilize a combination of study materials, such as textbooks, online resources, and practice exams. This will help you gain a comprehensive understanding of the material and expose you to different perspectives.
4. Engage in active learning: Instead of passively reading, try to actively engage with the material by taking notes, summarizing concepts, and teaching the material to someone else. This will help you retain information more effectively.
5. Practice, practice, practice: Use practice exams and questions to gauge your understanding and identify areas where you need improvement. Make sure to review the rationales for both correct and incorrect answers to reinforce your knowledge.
6. Join a study group: Connect with other candidates preparing for the CFRN exam. Sharing your knowledge, discussing concepts, and solving problems together can enhance your understanding and keep you motivated.

Test-taking Tips:

1. Arrive prepared: Arrive at the testing center early, well-rested, and with any required documentation. This will help you feel more relaxed and focused.
2. Manage your time: Keep an eye on the clock and pace yourself during the exam. Allocate enough time for each question, and avoid spending too much time on difficult questions.
3. Read the questions carefully: Make sure you understand what the question is asking before attempting to answer it. Look for keywords and phrases that may provide clues.
4. Eliminate incorrect answers: Use the process of elimination to narrow down your choices. Eliminate answers that are obviously incorrect, and then consider the remaining options.
5. Trust your instincts: If you're unsure about an answer, trust your first instinct. Avoid changing your answers unless you have a strong reason to believe your initial choice was incorrect.
6. Maintain a positive attitude: Stay confident and focused during the exam. If you encounter a challenging question, take a deep breath, relax, and give it your best shot.

Remember, adequate preparation, consistent practice, and a positive mindset are key factors in successfully tackling the CFRN exam. Good luck!

Practice Exam Section:

Welcome to the practice exam section! This part of the study guide has been designed to help you assess your understanding of the material and reinforce your learning. We believe that practice exams play a crucial role in preparing for the exam, allowing you to test your knowledge and get a feel for the types of questions you will encounter during the actual test. In fact, according to studies, one of the most important factors of success is practice questions. the more practice questions you take, the higher you score.

We have taken a unique approach in this section by providing the answer directly after each question. The rationale behind this decision is to prevent unnecessary page flipping, streamline your learning experience, and make it more efficient. By having the answers readily available, you can immediately review and understand the correct response without losing your train of thought or having to search through the guide. So make sure to hide the answer and prevent peaking by using paper or something of that manner.

This format encourages an interactive and engaging experience, allowing you to learn from any mistakes and reinforce your understanding of the concepts.

As you work through these practice questions, remember to stay focused, be patient with yourself, and use the answers as a learning tool to further solidify your knowledge. Good luck, and happy practicing!

1. A helicopter transporting a patient experiences a sudden decrease in cabin pressure at high altitude. Which of the following symptoms is most likely to occur in the patient as a result of the pressure change?
a) Hypoxia
b) Hyperventilation
c) Hypothermia
d) Hyperglycemia

Answer: a) Hypoxia
Explanation: At high altitudes, there is a reduction in atmospheric pressure and a decrease in the partial pressure of oxygen. This can lead to hypoxia, which is a deficiency in the amount of oxygen reaching the body's tissues. Hyperventilation, hypothermia, and hyperglycemia are not directly related to changes in cabin pressure at high altitude.

2. What is the primary purpose of using a pneumatic anti-shock garment (PASG) during patient transport?
a) To reduce pain from fractures
b) To maintain body temperature
c) To increase venous return and improve cardiac output
d) To prevent deep vein thrombosis

Answer: c) To increase venous return and improve cardiac output
Explanation: A pneumatic anti-shock garment (PASG) is an inflatable device that can be wrapped around the legs or lower abdomen to increase venous return and improve cardiac output in patients experiencing shock. It does not directly address pain, body temperature, or prevention of deep vein thrombosis.

3. Which of the following is the most important factor to consider when selecting an appropriate landing zone for a helicopter during a patient transport?
a) Proximity to a fuel source
b) Size and surface condition of the area
c) Availability of ground transportation
d) Weather conditions

Answer: b) Size and surface condition of the area
Explanation: The size and surface condition of the landing zone are crucial for the safety of the helicopter and crew. A suitable landing zone should be large enough, level, and free of obstructions or hazards. While proximity to a fuel source, availability of ground transportation, and weather conditions are also important considerations, the landing zone's suitability is paramount.

4. In an aeromedical transport situation, what is the main advantage of a fixed-wing aircraft compared to a helicopter?
a) Increased speed and range
b) Ability to land in confined spaces
c) Better maneuverability
d) Lower operational costs

Answer: a) Increased speed and range
Explanation: Fixed-wing aircraft have an advantage in speed and range compared to helicopters, allowing them to cover longer distances more quickly. While helicopters can land in confined spaces and are more maneuverable, fixed-wing aircraft are better suited for longer transport missions.

5. When assessing a patient's need for aeromedical transport, which of the following factors should be prioritized?
a) Patient's insurance coverage
b) Distance to the nearest hospital
c) Severity of the patient's condition
d) Availability of ground transport

Answer: c) Severity of the patient's condition
Explanation: The primary factor in determining the need for aeromedical transport is the severity of the patient's condition and the potential for improved outcomes with rapid transport to a specialized facility. While insurance coverage, distance to the nearest hospital, and availability of ground transport can all be considerations, the patient's condition and potential for improved care should be the top priority.

6. Which of the following physiological changes is most likely to occur in a patient during transport at high altitude?
a) Hypoxia
b) Hyperventilation
c) Hyperthermia
d) Hypoglycemia

Answer: a) Hypoxia
Explanation: At high altitudes, the partial pressure of oxygen decreases, which can lead to hypoxia or a deficiency in the amount of oxygen reaching the body's tissues. Hyperventilation, hyperthermia, and hypoglycemia are not directly related to altitude changes during transport.

7. During patient transport, excessive vibration can cause which of the following effects?
a) Increased patient comfort
b) Improved circulation
c) Fatigue and discomfort for the patient
d) Enhanced oxygen delivery

Answer: c) Fatigue and discomfort for the patient
Explanation: Excessive vibration during transport can cause fatigue, discomfort, and exacerbate pain for the patient. It does not improve patient comfort, circulation, or oxygen delivery.

8. What is the primary reason for temperature regulation during patient transport?
a) To prevent hypothermia or hyperthermia
b) To reduce patient anxiety
c) To maintain equipment functionality
d) To comply with regulations

Answer: a) To prevent hypothermia or hyperthermia
Explanation: The main goal of temperature regulation during patient transport is to prevent hypothermia or hyperthermia, both of which can have detrimental effects on the patient's condition. While reducing patient anxiety, maintaining equipment functionality, and complying with regulations are also important, the patient's well-being is the primary concern.

9. How can noise levels during patient transport impact patient care?
a) They can interfere with communication among the medical team
b) They can cause motion sickness
c) They can trigger allergic reactions
d) They can lead to rapid dehydration

Answer: a) They can interfere with communication among the medical team
Explanation: High noise levels during patient transport can interfere with communication among the medical team, potentially compromising patient care. Noise levels do not directly cause motion sickness, trigger allergic reactions, or lead to rapid dehydration.

10. In the context of transport physiology, what is the primary concern regarding the effects of altitude on a patient with a pneumothorax?
a) Increased intracranial pressure
b) Decreased respiratory rate
c) Expansion of trapped gas within the pleural space
d) Reduced blood pressure

Answer: c) Expansion of trapped gas within the pleural space
Explanation: During transport at high altitude, the primary concern for a patient with a pneumothorax is the expansion of trapped gas within the pleural space due to decreased atmospheric pressure. This can worsen the pneumothorax and potentially lead to a life-threatening tension pneumothorax. The other options do not directly relate to the effects of altitude on a patient with a pneumothorax.

11. What is the primary purpose of crew resource management (CRM) in a transport setting?
a) To establish a hierarchy among team members
b) To improve decision-making and communication among the crew
c) To reduce the workload of individual team members
d) To ensure that all equipment is functioning properly

Answer: b) To improve decision-making and communication among the crew
Explanation: Crew resource management (CRM) is designed to improve decision-making and communication among the crew to enhance patient care and safety. While CRM may indirectly impact workload and equipment management, its primary focus is on teamwork and communication.

12. In the event of an emergency landing, which of the following actions should be prioritized to improve survival chances?
a) Locating and using the aircraft's first aid kit
b) Ensuring proper communication with air traffic control
c) Performing a risk assessment of the surrounding environment
d) Securing all loose objects and preparing for impact

Answer: d) Securing all loose objects and preparing for impact
Explanation: In an emergency landing situation, securing all loose objects and preparing for impact is crucial to minimize the risk of injury and improve the chances of survival. While the other options may be relevant in different scenarios, they are not the priority in an emergency landing situation.

13. What is one key aspect of vehicle safety during patient transport?
a) Maintaining a consistent speed at all times
b) Using lights and sirens only when necessary
c) Driving aggressively to shorten transport time
d) Leaving doors unlocked for quick patient access

Answer: b) Using lights and sirens only when necessary
Explanation: Using lights and sirens only when necessary helps to minimize the risk of accidents, as excessive use can lead to traffic confusion and increased risk of collisions. The other options can increase the risk of accidents and compromise safety.

14. What is an important consideration when selecting a landing zone for a medical helicopter?
a) Proximity to a body of water
b) Availability of a large, flat, and unobstructed area
c) The amount of vegetation in the area
d) The presence of wildlife

Answer: b) Availability of a large, flat, and unobstructed area
Explanation: When selecting a landing zone for a medical helicopter, it is important to choose a large, flat, and unobstructed area to minimize the risk of accidents during landing and takeoff. Proximity to water, vegetation, and wildlife are not the primary considerations for landing zone selection.

15. Which of the following is an essential skill for transport medical personnel to possess in case of an emergency situation in a remote area?
a) Ability to repair damaged equipment
b) Knowledge of basic survival skills
c) Expertise in tracking weather patterns
d) Fluency in multiple languages

Answer: b) Knowledge of basic survival skills
Explanation: In an emergency situation in a remote area, it is crucial for transport medical personnel to possess basic survival skills, such as finding shelter, starting a fire, and signaling for help. While the other skills listed may be useful in certain scenarios, they are not as vital for survival in a remote emergency situation.

16. When transporting a patient with suspected spinal injury, which of the following is the most appropriate positioning?
a) Supine with the head elevated
b) In the recovery position
c) Spine immobilized on a long spine board
d) Sitting up with a cervical collar

Answer: c) Spine immobilized on a long spine board
Explanation: When a spinal injury is suspected, it is crucial to immobilize the patient's spine to prevent further injury. The most appropriate positioning for this is on a long spine board with cervical spine protection.

17. What is a primary consideration when managing medical equipment during patient transport?
a) Ensuring all equipment is turned off to save battery life
b) Regularly checking equipment for proper functioning and securement
c) Utilizing multiple devices for redundancy
d) Keeping all equipment stored in a single location

Answer: b) Regularly checking equipment for proper functioning and securement
Explanation: During patient transport, it is essential to regularly check medical equipment for proper functioning and securement to ensure patient safety and effective treatment. The other options listed do not prioritize patient safety and effective treatment.

18. When transporting a patient experiencing respiratory distress, what is an essential intervention?
a) Administering supplemental oxygen as needed
b) Immediately sedating the patient
c) Positioning the patient in a prone position
d) Restricting fluids during transport

Answer: a) Administering supplemental oxygen as needed
Explanation: In cases of respiratory distress, providing supplemental oxygen is essential to maintain adequate oxygen levels and support respiratory function. The other options listed do not directly address the patient's respiratory needs.

19. Which of the following actions should be taken if a patient experiences a sudden change in condition during transport?
a) Continue with the original transport plan
b) Stop the transport and wait for additional help
c) Reassess the patient and modify treatment as needed
d) Contact the patient's primary care physician for advice

Answer: c) Reassess the patient and modify treatment as needed
Explanation: If a patient experiences a sudden change in condition during transport, it is crucial to reassess the patient and modify treatment as needed to address the new situation. The other options do not prioritize the patient's immediate needs.

20. What is a key factor to consider when preparing a patient for transport with an intravenous (IV) infusion?
a) Securing the IV site and monitoring for complications
b) Hanging multiple IV bags for redundancy
c) Administering the entire infusion before transport
d) Elevating the patient's arm to reduce blood flow

Answer: a) Securing the IV site and monitoring for complications
Explanation: When preparing a patient for transport with an IV infusion, it is important to secure the IV site and monitor for complications such as infiltration, phlebitis, or occlusion. The other options do not address patient safety and the effective management of the IV infusion during transport.

21. Which of the following is a key component of patient rights according to the Health Insurance Portability and Accountability Act (HIPAA)?
a) The right to access their medical records
b) The right to refuse treatment without explanation
c) The right to demand specific medications
d) The right to choose their healthcare provider during an emergency

Answer: a) The right to access their medical records
Explanation: HIPAA establishes patient rights, including the right to access their medical records. The other options listed are not specifically mentioned in the HIPAA regulations.

22. When obtaining informed consent from a patient, which of the following is NOT a necessary element to discuss?
a) The potential risks of the treatment
b) The benefits of the treatment
c) Alternative treatment options
d) The patient's financial status

Answer: d) The patient's financial status
Explanation: Informed consent involves discussing the potential risks, benefits, and alternative options related to the treatment. The patient's financial status is not a necessary element for informed consent.

23. In what situation is it appropriate to breach patient confidentiality in flight nursing?
a) When the patient's family members ask for an update
b) When discussing the patient's condition with a colleague during a break
c) When reporting suspected child abuse
d) When discussing the case on social media without using the patient's name

Answer: c) When reporting suspected child abuse
Explanation: Breaching patient confidentiality is only appropriate when there is a legal or ethical obligation to do so, such as reporting suspected child abuse. The other situations listed are not appropriate instances to disclose patient information.

24. Which of the following is considered an ethical principle in healthcare?
a) Beneficence
b) Personal bias
c) Financial gain
d) Hierarchy

Answer: a) Beneficence
Explanation: Beneficence is an ethical principle in healthcare that focuses on promoting the well-being of patients and taking actions that benefit them. The other options listed are not considered ethical principles in healthcare.

25. What is the primary purpose of documenting patient care during a transport?
a) To protect the healthcare provider in case of legal action
b) To communicate the patient's condition and treatment to other healthcare providers
c) To track the healthcare provider's performance metrics
d) To obtain reimbursement from insurance companies

Answer: b) To communicate the patient's condition and treatment to other healthcare providers
Explanation: The primary purpose of documentation is to communicate the patient's condition, treatment, and any changes that occurred during transport to other healthcare providers involved in the patient's care. The other options listed may be secondary benefits of documentation but are not the primary purpose.

26. A patient presenting with wheezing, shortness of breath, and a history of asthma is most likely experiencing:
a) Pulmonary edema
b) Pneumothorax
c) Bronchospasm
d) Pulmonary embolism

Answer: c) Bronchospasm
Explanation: Wheezing, shortness of breath, and a history of asthma are typical signs of a bronchospasm, which is a constriction of the airways often seen in asthma patients. The other options are less likely given the patient's symptoms and history.

27. Which of the following is the primary initial treatment for a patient with a suspected tension pneumothorax?
a) Administering supplemental oxygen
b) Performing needle decompression
c) Initiating positive pressure ventilation
d) Administering bronchodilators

Answer: b) Performing needle decompression
Explanation: Needle decompression is the primary initial treatment for a suspected tension pneumothorax, as it relieves pressure in the pleural space and allows the lung to re-expand. The other options may be appropriate for other respiratory emergencies but are not the primary treatments for tension pneumothorax.

28. What is the most common cause of acute respiratory distress syndrome (ARDS)?
a) Chronic obstructive pulmonary disease (COPD)
b) Sepsis
c) Asthma
d) Pulmonary embolism

Answer: b) Sepsis
Explanation: Sepsis is the most common cause of ARDS, a severe lung condition characterized by rapid onset of widespread inflammation in the lungs. The other options may contribute to respiratory distress but are not the most common causes of ARDS.

29. A patient with sudden shortness of breath, chest pain, and low oxygen saturation is likely experiencing:
a) Acute asthma exacerbation
b) Pneumonia
c) Pulmonary embolism
d) Congestive heart failure

Answer: c) Pulmonary embolism
Explanation: Sudden onset of shortness of breath, chest pain, and low oxygen saturation are classic signs of a pulmonary embolism, which occurs when a blood clot blocks one or more arteries in the lungs. The other options may cause respiratory distress but are less likely given the patient's symptoms.

30. Which of the following medications is most appropriate for treating a moderate asthma exacerbation?
a) Epinephrine
b) Albuterol
c) Furosemide
d) Nitroglycerin

Answer: b) Albuterol
Explanation: Albuterol, a short-acting beta-agonist, is the most appropriate medication for treating a moderate asthma exacerbation, as it helps to relax the smooth muscles in the airways, improving airflow. The other medications listed are not the first-line treatments for moderate asthma exacerbations.

31. Which of the following airway adjuncts is most appropriate for a patient with an intact gag reflex?
a) Oropharyngeal airway (OPA)
b) Nasopharyngeal airway (NPA)
c) Laryngeal mask airway (LMA)
d) Endotracheal tube (ETT)

Answer: b) Nasopharyngeal airway (NPA)
Explanation: An NPA is most appropriate for patients with an intact gag reflex, as it can be inserted without stimulating the gag reflex. The other options are generally better suited for patients with a diminished or absent gag reflex.

32. In which of the following situations is a cricothyrotomy most likely indicated?
a) Upper airway obstruction due to foreign body
b) Severe facial trauma with airway compromise
c) Pneumothorax with respiratory distress
d) Acute asthma exacerbation unresponsive to treatment

Answer: b) Severe facial trauma with airway compromise
Explanation: A cricothyrotomy is a surgical airway procedure that is most likely indicated in cases of severe facial trauma with airway compromise when other airway management techniques have failed or are not feasible.

33. The most common complication of endotracheal intubation is:
a) Esophageal intubation
b) Dental injury
c) Laryngospasm
d) Hypoxia

Answer: a) Esophageal intubation
Explanation: Esophageal intubation is the most common complication of endotracheal intubation. It occurs when the endotracheal tube is inadvertently placed into the esophagus instead of the trachea, which can lead to inadequate ventilation and potential harm to the patient.

34. When using a laryngeal mask airway (LMA), it is important to:
a) Inflate the cuff until the pilot balloon is firm
b) Insert the device without the use of a laryngoscope
c) Perform a Sellick maneuver during insertion
d) Confirm proper placement with a capnography device

Answer: b) Insert the device without the use of a laryngoscope
Explanation: An LMA is designed to be inserted blindly without the use of a laryngoscope. The other options listed are not accurate or appropriate when using an LMA for airway management.

35. A patient is being ventilated with a bag-valve-mask (BVM) device. Despite a good mask seal and adequate chest rise, the patient's oxygen saturation remains low. What should be considered as a potential cause?
a) The patient may require endotracheal intubation
b) The BVM device may be malfunctioning
c) The patient may have a tension pneumothorax
d) The oxygen flow rate is too low

Answer: c) The patient may have a tension pneumothorax
Explanation: A tension pneumothorax can cause low oxygen saturation despite adequate BVM ventilation, as it impairs gas exchange in the lungs. In such cases, needle decompression or chest tube insertion may be required. The other options may be relevant in different situations, but a tension pneumothorax should be considered and ruled out first.

36. Which mode of mechanical ventilation provides a set tidal volume with each breath and allows the patient to initiate additional breaths?
a) Assist-Control (AC) ventilation
b) Synchronized Intermittent Mandatory Ventilation (SIMV)
c) Pressure Support Ventilation (PSV)
d) Continuous Positive Airway Pressure (CPAP)

Answer: b) Synchronized Intermittent Mandatory Ventilation (SIMV)
Explanation: SIMV delivers a set tidal volume with each mandatory breath and allows the patient to initiate additional spontaneous breaths. The other modes listed have different characteristics and functions.

37. Non-invasive positive pressure ventilation (NIPPV) is most appropriate for which of the following patient presentations?
a) Acute respiratory distress with an altered mental status
b) Severe facial trauma with compromised airway
c) Acute exacerbation of chronic obstructive pulmonary disease (COPD)
d) Massive hemoptysis

Answer: c) Acute exacerbation of chronic obstructive pulmonary disease (COPD)
Explanation: NIPPV is most appropriate for patients with an acute exacerbation of COPD, as it can improve oxygenation and ventilation without the need for invasive airway management. The other options may require alternative interventions or more invasive airway management.

38. Which of the following complications is most commonly associated with mechanical ventilation?
a) Pneumothorax
b) Ventilator-associated pneumonia
c) Pulmonary edema
d) Airway trauma

Answer: b) Ventilator-associated pneumonia
Explanation: Ventilator-associated pneumonia is a common complication associated with mechanical ventilation. The other complications listed can also occur but are less common.

39. A patient receiving mechanical ventilation begins to exhibit signs of increased intrathoracic pressure. Which ventilator adjustment is most appropriate to reduce this pressure?
a) Increase tidal volume
b) Decrease respiratory rate
c) Decrease inspiratory time
d) Increase positive end-expiratory pressure (PEEP)

Answer: c) Decrease inspiratory time
Explanation: Decreasing inspiratory time can help reduce intrathoracic pressure, as it allows for more time for exhalation and prevents breath stacking. The other adjustments listed may not effectively address increased intrathoracic pressure.

40. Which of the following conditions is an indication for the use of continuous positive airway pressure (CPAP) in a spontaneously breathing patient?
a) Acute respiratory failure with a compromised airway
b) Acute pulmonary edema
c) Massive hemoptysis
d) Obstructive sleep apnea

Answer: b) Acute pulmonary edema
Explanation: CPAP can be used to manage acute pulmonary edema in spontaneously breathing patients, as it helps to improve oxygenation and reduce the work of breathing. The other conditions listed may require alternative interventions or more invasive airway management.

41. A patient presents with sudden onset of dyspnea, pleuritic chest pain, and decreased breath sounds on one side. The most likely diagnosis is:
a) Asthma
b) Chronic obstructive pulmonary disease (COPD)
c) Pulmonary embolism
d) Pneumothorax

Answer: d) Pneumothorax
Explanation: The sudden onset of dyspnea, pleuritic chest pain, and decreased breath sounds on one side are characteristic of a pneumothorax. The other options have different presentations and symptoms.

42. A patient with a history of COPD presents with increased shortness of breath, wheezing, and a productive cough. Which medication is most appropriate for initial treatment?
a) Inhaled short-acting beta-agonist (SABA)
b) Inhaled corticosteroid
c) Oral antibiotic
d) Intravenous diuretic

Answer: a) Inhaled short-acting beta-agonist (SABA)
Explanation: An inhaled SABA is the first-line treatment for acute exacerbations of COPD, as it helps to relieve bronchospasm and improve airflow. The other medications may be used in specific circumstances or as adjuncts to treatment.

43. Which of the following signs is most indicative of a pulmonary embolism?
a) Unilateral leg swelling
b) Barrel-shaped chest
c) Prolonged expiration
d) Decreased tactile fremitus

Answer: a) Unilateral leg swelling
Explanation: Unilateral leg swelling is a common sign of deep vein thrombosis (DVT), which can lead to a pulmonary embolism. The other options are more characteristic of different respiratory conditions.

44. In a patient with suspected tension pneumothorax, which of the following findings is most likely to be observed?
a) Hyperresonance to percussion on the affected side
b) Tracheal deviation away from the affected side
c) Decreased breath sounds on the affected side
d) All of the above

Answer: d) All of the above
Explanation: All of the listed findings are characteristic of tension pneumothorax, which is a life-threatening condition requiring immediate intervention.

45. A patient with a known history of asthma presents with a sudden, severe asthma attack. Initial treatment with a short-acting beta-agonist is not providing relief. What is the next appropriate intervention?
a) Administer inhaled corticosteroids
b) Initiate non-invasive positive pressure ventilation (NIPPV)
c) Administer intravenous magnesium sulfate
d) Administer epinephrine

Answer: c) Administer intravenous magnesium sulfate
Explanation: Intravenous magnesium sulfate can be used as an adjunct treatment in severe asthma attacks that do not respond to initial treatment with short-acting beta-agonists. The other interventions may be considered, but magnesium sulfate is the preferred next step in this scenario.

46. A patient presents with sudden onset of severe chest pain, diaphoresis, and shortness of breath. The 12-lead ECG reveals ST-segment elevation in leads V2-V4. What is the most likely diagnosis?
a) Acute pericarditis
b) Anterior wall myocardial infarction (MI)
c) Aortic dissection
d) Pulmonary embolism

Answer: b) Anterior wall myocardial infarction (MI)
Explanation: The patient's symptoms and ST-segment elevation in leads V2-V4 are consistent with an anterior wall MI. The other options have different ECG findings and clinical presentations.

47. A patient with a history of hypertension presents with tearing chest pain radiating to the back. Which diagnostic test is most appropriate to confirm the suspected diagnosis?
a) 12-lead ECG
b) Chest X-ray
c) CT angiography
d) Echocardiogram

Answer: c) CT angiography
Explanation: The patient's symptoms are suggestive of aortic dissection, and a CT angiography is the most appropriate test to confirm the diagnosis. The other tests may be used to evaluate different cardiovascular conditions.

48. Which medication is the preferred initial treatment for a patient with unstable angina?
a) Morphine
b) Nitroglycerin
c) Aspirin
d) Beta-blocker

Answer: c) Aspirin
Explanation: Aspirin is the preferred initial treatment for unstable angina, as it inhibits platelet aggregation and reduces the risk of MI. The other medications may be used as adjuncts or in specific circumstances.

49. A patient with congestive heart failure presents with worsening dyspnea and peripheral edema. Which intervention is most appropriate?
a) Administer a loop diuretic
b) Initiate non-invasive positive pressure ventilation (NIPPV)
c) Administer intravenous nitroglycerin
d) Administer a beta-blocker

Answer: a) Administer a loop diuretic
Explanation: A loop diuretic is the most appropriate intervention for a patient with congestive heart failure presenting with worsening symptoms, as it helps to remove excess fluid and reduce the workload on the heart. The other interventions may be considered, but a loop diuretic is the preferred initial treatment.

50. A patient presents with ventricular fibrillation. Which of the following interventions should be performed first?
a) Administer amiodarone
b) Perform immediate defibrillation
c) Begin CPR
d) Administer epinephrine

Answer: b) Perform immediate defibrillation
Explanation: Immediate defibrillation is the first intervention for ventricular fibrillation, as it can potentially restore a normal cardiac rhythm. The other interventions may be used in the advanced cardiac life support (ACLS) algorithm if defibrillation is unsuccessful.

51. A patient presents with palpitations and dizziness. The ECG reveals a regular, narrow complex tachycardia with a heart rate of 180 beats per minute. What is the most likely diagnosis?
a) Sinus tachycardia
b) Atrial fibrillation
c) Supraventricular tachycardia (SVT)
d) Ventricular tachycardia

Answer: c) Supraventricular tachycardia (SVT)
Explanation: The ECG findings of a regular, narrow complex tachycardia with a heart rate around 180 bpm are consistent with SVT. The other options have different ECG findings and clinical presentations.

52. Which ECG lead is most commonly used for continuous cardiac monitoring in patients with suspected acute coronary syndrome?
a) Lead I
b) Lead II
c) Lead V1
d) Lead V5

Answer: b) Lead II
Explanation: Lead II is most commonly used for continuous cardiac monitoring in patients with suspected acute coronary syndrome because it provides a clear view of the P, QRS, and T waves, and is sensitive to detecting ST-segment changes.

53. A patient with a history of myocardial infarction presents with chest pain. The ECG shows ST-segment depression and T-wave inversion in leads V4-V6. What is the most likely diagnosis?
a) Anterior wall myocardial ischemia
b) Posterior wall myocardial ischemia
c) Lateral wall myocardial ischemia
d) Inferior wall myocardial ischemia

Answer: c) Lateral wall myocardial ischemia
Explanation: ST-segment depression and T-wave inversion in leads V4-V6 are indicative of lateral wall myocardial ischemia. The other options would have different ECG findings.

54. A patient presents with an irregularly irregular rhythm and a heart rate of 150 bpm on the ECG. What is the most likely diagnosis?
a) Atrial fibrillation with rapid ventricular response
b) Atrial flutter
c) Supraventricular tachycardia
d) Ventricular fibrillation

Answer: a) Atrial fibrillation with rapid ventricular response
Explanation: The ECG findings of an irregularly irregular rhythm and a heart rate of 150 bpm are consistent with atrial fibrillation with rapid ventricular response. The other options have different ECG findings and clinical presentations.

55. In a patient with a suspected acute myocardial infarction, which of the following interventions should be performed first?
a) Administer nitroglycerin
b) Obtain a 12-lead ECG
c) Administer morphine
d) Administer aspirin

Answer: b) Obtain a 12-lead ECG
Explanation: Obtaining a 12-lead ECG is the first intervention for a patient with a suspected acute myocardial infarction, as it helps to confirm the diagnosis and guide further treatment. The other interventions can be performed afterward based on the ECG findings and the patient's clinical presentation.

56. Which of the following is the preferred vascular access method for fluid resuscitation in a hemodynamically unstable patient when peripheral intravenous access cannot be obtained?
a) Central venous access
b) Intraosseous access
c) Peripherally inserted central catheter (PICC)
d) Umbilical venous catheter

Answer: b) Intraosseous access
Explanation: Intraosseous access is the preferred method for fluid resuscitation in a hemodynamically unstable patient when peripheral intravenous access is not possible, as it provides rapid access to the systemic circulation and allows for the administration of fluids and medications.

57. Which type of fluid is typically used for the initial resuscitation of a patient in septic shock?
a) Crystalloid solution
b) Colloid solution
c) Hypertonic saline
d) Packed red blood cells

Answer: a) Crystalloid solution
Explanation: Crystalloid solutions, such as normal saline or lactated Ringer's solution, are typically used for the initial resuscitation of a patient in septic shock because they rapidly expand the intravascular volume and improve tissue perfusion.

58. In which anatomical location is the tip of a properly placed central venous catheter usually positioned?
a) Right atrium
b) Superior vena cava
c) Inferior vena cava
d) Subclavian vein

Answer: b) Superior vena cava
Explanation: The tip of a properly placed central venous catheter should be positioned in the superior vena cava, just above the right atrium, to ensure optimal delivery of fluids and medications and to minimize the risk of complications.

59. When placing a peripheral intravenous catheter, what is the recommended angle of needle insertion relative to the skin?
a) 10-15 degrees
b) 25-30 degrees
c) 45-60 degrees
d) 75-90 degrees

Answer: a) 10-15 degrees
Explanation: When placing a peripheral intravenous catheter, the recommended angle of needle insertion relative to the skin is 10-15 degrees, as this angle provides the best chance of accessing the vein without puncturing through the opposite wall.

60. What is the primary goal of fluid resuscitation in a patient with hypovolemic shock?
a) Increase blood pressure
b) Improve tissue oxygenation
c) Restore intravascular volume
d) Correct electrolyte imbalances

Answer: c) Restore intravascular volume
Explanation: The primary goal of fluid resuscitation in a patient with hypovolemic shock is to restore intravascular volume, which will subsequently improve tissue perfusion, blood pressure, and oxygenation.

61. What is the primary mechanism of action of vasopressor medications in the treatment of shock?
a) Vasodilation of arterial vessels
b) Increasing myocardial contractility
c) Vasoconstriction of arterial vessels
d) Increasing heart rate

Answer: c) Vasoconstriction of arterial vessels
Explanation: Vasopressor medications, such as norepinephrine and epinephrine, primarily act by causing vasoconstriction of arterial vessels, which increases systemic vascular resistance and improves blood pressure in patients with shock.

62. Which of the following antiarrhythmic medications is commonly used for the acute management of supraventricular tachycardia (SVT)?
a) Amiodarone
b) Lidocaine
c) Adenosine
d) Digoxin

Answer: c) Adenosine
Explanation: Adenosine is a short-acting antiarrhythmic medication that is commonly used for the acute management of supraventricular tachycardia (SVT) due to its ability to temporarily block conduction through the atrioventricular (AV) node, potentially restoring normal sinus rhythm.

63. When administering a heparin infusion for anticoagulation, what laboratory value is most commonly used to monitor the therapeutic effect?
a) International normalized ratio (INR)
b) Prothrombin time (PT)
c) Activated partial thromboplastin time (aPTT)
d) Platelet count

Answer: c) Activated partial thromboplastin time (aPTT)
Explanation: The activated partial thromboplastin time (aPTT) is the most commonly used laboratory value to monitor the therapeutic effect of a heparin infusion, as it provides a measure of the anticoagulant effect and helps guide adjustments in the infusion rate.

64. Which of the following medications is a calcium channel blocker commonly used for rate control in atrial fibrillation?
a) Metoprolol
b) Diltiazem
c) Amiodarone
d) Flecainide

Answer: b) Diltiazem
Explanation: Diltiazem is a calcium channel blocker that is commonly used for rate control in atrial fibrillation, as it slows conduction through the atrioventricular (AV) node and reduces the ventricular response rate.

65. In a patient with a systolic blood pressure of 70 mmHg and signs of poor perfusion, which of the following vasopressor medications would be the most appropriate initial choice?
a) Dopamine
b) Norepinephrine
c) Epinephrine
d) Phenylephrine

Answer: b) Norepinephrine
Explanation: Norepinephrine is the most appropriate initial choice for a patient with a systolic blood pressure of 70 mmHg and signs of poor perfusion, as it is a potent vasoconstrictor that effectively increases systemic vascular resistance and blood pressure in patients with shock.

66. In a patient with a suspected tension pneumothorax, which of the following signs is most suggestive of this life-threatening condition?
a) Decreased breath sounds on the affected side
b) Tracheal deviation away from the affected side
c) Jugular venous distention
d) Hypotension

Answer: b) Tracheal deviation away from the affected side
Explanation: Tracheal deviation away from the affected side is a late and ominous sign of tension pneumothorax, indicating increased intrathoracic pressure and potential compression of the mediastinal structures, which can lead to rapid cardiovascular collapse.

67. Which of the following is the most common cause of status epilepticus in adults?
a) Traumatic brain injury
b) Hypoglycemia
c) Stroke
d) Withdrawal from alcohol or benzodiazepines

Answer: d) Withdrawal from alcohol or benzodiazepines
Explanation: Withdrawal from alcohol or benzodiazepines is the most common cause of status epilepticus in adults, as the sudden cessation of these substances can lead to severe and potentially life-threatening seizures.

68. A patient presenting with altered mental status, hyperthermia, and muscle rigidity should be evaluated for which life-threatening condition?
a) Serotonin syndrome
b) Neuroleptic malignant syndrome
c) Malignant hyperthermia
d) Heat stroke

Answer: b) Neuroleptic malignant syndrome. Explanation: Neuroleptic malignant syndrome is a life-threatening condition characterized by altered mental status, hyperthermia, and muscle rigidity, typically occurring as a result of exposure to antipsychotic medications or other dopamine antagonists.

69. A patient with a suspected snakebite from a venomous snake presents with severe pain, swelling, and ecchymosis at the bite site. What is the most appropriate initial management?
a) Apply a tourniquet proximal to the bite site
b) Immobilize the affected extremity and keep it at heart level
c) Administer antivenom immediately
d) Apply ice to the bite site

Answer: b) Immobilize the affected extremity and keep it at heart level. Explanation: Immobilizing the affected extremity and keeping it at heart level can help minimize venom spread and reduce the risk of systemic effects. Tourniquets, ice, and immediate antivenom administration are not recommended as initial management for most venomous snakebites.

70. In a patient with a suspected spinal cord injury, which of the following interventions is the highest priority?
a) Administering high-flow oxygen
b) Performing a rapid trauma assessment
c) Immobilizing the spine with a cervical collar and backboard
d) Establishing intravenous access

Answer: c) Immobilizing the spine with a cervical collar and backboard
Explanation: In a patient with a suspected spinal cord injury, the highest priority is immobilizing the spine with a cervical collar and backboard to prevent further damage to the spinal cord. Other interventions, such as oxygen administration, trauma assessment, and intravenous access, are also important but should be performed after spinal immobilization.

71. A patient with type 1 diabetes presents with polyuria, polydipsia, and rapid, deep respirations. Which of the following laboratory findings is most consistent with the suspected diagnosis of diabetic ketoacidosis (DKA)?
a) Low serum glucose
b) High serum bicarbonate
c) High serum potassium
d) Low serum osmolality

Answer: c) High serum potassium
Explanation: In DKA, serum potassium levels are typically elevated due to acidosis and extracellular shifts of potassium. The other options are not consistent with DKA, as patients usually have high serum glucose, low serum bicarbonate, and high serum osmolality.

72. A patient presents with severe headache, stiff neck, and photophobia. Which of the following is the most appropriate initial management for this patient with suspected bacterial meningitis?
a) Immediate lumbar puncture
b) Administration of broad-spectrum antibiotics
c) Initiation of antiviral therapy
d) Non-contrast head CT scan

Answer: b) Administration of broad-spectrum antibiotics
Explanation: In a patient with suspected bacterial meningitis, the administration of broad-spectrum antibiotics should not be delayed, as early treatment can significantly improve outcomes. A lumbar puncture or imaging may be performed after initiating antibiotics.

73. A patient with a history of chronic kidney disease presents with shortness of breath, hypertension, and pulmonary crackles. Which of the following interventions is most appropriate for this patient with suspected volume overload?
a) Administration of a loop diuretic
b) Hemodialysis
c) Intravenous fluid resuscitation
d) Administration of an inotropic agent

Answer: a) Administration of a loop diuretic

Explanation: In patients with suspected volume overload due to chronic kidney disease, administration of a loop diuretic can help remove excess fluid and alleviate symptoms. Hemodialysis may be considered if diuretics are ineffective, while fluid resuscitation and inotropic agents are not appropriate in this context.

74. A patient presents with altered mental status, diaphoresis, and tremors. Blood glucose is 40 mg/dL. What is the most appropriate initial intervention?
a) Administration of intravenous dextrose
b) Administration of subcutaneous insulin
c) Administration of oral glucose gel
d) Administration of glucagon

Answer: a) Administration of intravenous dextrose. Explanation: In a patient with severe hypoglycemia and altered mental status, the most appropriate initial intervention is the administration of intravenous dextrose to rapidly raise blood glucose levels. Oral glucose gel and glucagon can be considered in patients with mild hypoglycemia who are awake and able to protect their airway.

75. Which of the following is the most common cause of upper gastrointestinal bleeding in adults?
a) Esophageal varices
b) Peptic ulcer disease
c) Mallory-Weiss tear
d) Gastric cancer

Answer: b) Peptic ulcer disease. Explanation: Peptic ulcer disease is the most common cause of upper gastrointestinal bleeding in adults. Other causes, such as esophageal varices, Mallory-Weiss tear, and gastric cancer, are less common but still significant contributors to upper gastrointestinal bleeding.

76. Which of the following is the most appropriate initial treatment for a patient with moderate hypothermia?
a) Active external rewarming with warm blankets
b) Passive external rewarming with dry clothing
c) Administration of warmed intravenous fluids
d) Immersion in warm water

Answer: b) Passive external rewarming with dry clothing. Explanation: In cases of moderate hypothermia, the most appropriate initial treatment is passive external rewarming, which involves removing wet clothing and replacing it with dry, insulated clothing or blankets. Active rewarming is more appropriate for severe hypothermia, while warmed intravenous fluids and immersion in warm water may also be considered for severe cases.

77. A hiker presents with headache, nausea, and difficulty walking after ascending a high-altitude mountain too quickly. What is the most appropriate treatment for this patient with suspected acute mountain sickness (AMS)?
a) Immediate descent to a lower altitude
b) Oxygen therapy
c) Acetazolamide administration
d) IV fluid administration

Answer: a) Immediate descent to a lower altitude
Explanation: The most appropriate treatment for AMS is to immediately descend to a lower altitude, as symptoms usually resolve with descent. Oxygen therapy and acetazolamide may be considered to alleviate symptoms, but descent should not be delayed. IV fluid administration is not indicated for AMS.

78. A patient presents with signs of severe dehydration, fever, and altered mental status after prolonged exposure to high temperatures. Which of the following conditions is most likely?
a) Heat exhaustion
b) Heat stroke
c) Heat cramps
d) Heat syncope

Answer: b) Heat stroke. Explanation: Heat stroke is characterized by severe dehydration, fever, and altered mental status after prolonged exposure to high temperatures. It is a life-threatening emergency that requires aggressive cooling measures. Heat exhaustion, heat cramps, and heat syncope are less severe heat-related illnesses with different presenting symptoms.

79. Which of the following is the most appropriate treatment for a patient with a mild case of frostbite?
a) Rapid rewarming in warm water
b) Slow rewarming with warm blankets
c) Massage the affected area
d) Application of dry heat

Answer: a) Rapid rewarming in warm water. Explanation: Rapid rewarming in warm water (40-42°C) is the most appropriate treatment for frostbite, as it helps to quickly restore blood flow and minimize tissue damage. Slow rewarming, massaging the affected area, and applying dry heat are not recommended for frostbite management.

80. A patient is found submerged in cold water and is unresponsive. Which of the following should be prioritized in the initial management of this suspected drowning victim?
a) Providing high-flow oxygen
b) Performing chest compressions
c) Performing rescue breaths
d) Immediate rewarming

Answer: c) Performing rescue breaths. Explanation: In the initial management of a suspected drowning victim, rescue breaths should be prioritized, as hypoxia is the primary cause of morbidity and mortality in drowning cases. Providing high-flow oxygen, chest compressions, and rewarming are important aspects of management, but rescue breaths should be initiated first.

81. A patient presents with a suspected tension pneumothorax. Which of the following interventions should be performed immediately?
a) Administration of oxygen
b) Needle decompression
c) Chest tube insertion
d) Emergency thoracotomy

Answer: b) Needle decompression

Explanation: In cases of suspected tension pneumothorax, immediate needle decompression is the most appropriate intervention to relieve the pressure and prevent further complications. Administration of oxygen, chest tube insertion, and emergency thoracotomy may be considered later in the management of the patient's condition.

82. A patient with a suspected cervical spine injury is being transported. What is the best method to maintain spinal immobilization during transport?
a) Cervical collar only
b) Cervical collar and rigid backboard
c) Logroll technique
d) Manual in-line stabilization

Answer: b) Cervical collar and rigid backboard

Explanation: A cervical collar in combination with a rigid backboard is the best method to maintain spinal immobilization during transport for patients with suspected cervical spine injuries. The logroll technique and manual in-line stabilization can be used during patient movement, but they do not provide the necessary immobilization during transport.

83. In a patient with a severe traumatic brain injury, which of the following should be the primary goal for managing intracranial pressure (ICP)?
a) Maintaining an ICP below 20 mmHg
b) Maintaining an ICP below 30 mmHg
c) Maintaining an ICP below 40 mmHg
d) Maintaining an ICP below 50 mmHg

Answer: a) Maintaining an ICP below 20 mmHg

Explanation: In patients with severe traumatic brain injury, the primary goal for managing ICP is to maintain it below 20 mmHg, as higher levels are associated with increased morbidity and mortality. Management may include sedation, paralysis, and osmotic therapy, among other interventions.

84. A patient has sustained a significant burn injury. What is the most appropriate fluid resuscitation strategy for this patient during the first 24 hours?
a) Lactated Ringer's solution
b) Normal saline
c) 5% dextrose in water
d) Hypertonic saline

Answer: a) Lactated Ringer's solution

Explanation: The most appropriate fluid resuscitation strategy for burn patients during the first 24 hours is Lactated Ringer's solution, following the Parkland formula. Normal saline, 5% dextrose in water, and hypertonic saline are not typically used for initial fluid resuscitation in burn patients.

84. Which of the following is the most appropriate initial treatment for an open fracture?
a) Immediate reduction and splinting
b) Application of a tourniquet
c) Administration of intravenous antibiotics
d) Immediate surgical intervention

Answer: c) Administration of intravenous antibiotics
Explanation: The most appropriate initial treatment for an open fracture is administration of intravenous antibiotics to prevent infection. Immediate reduction, splinting, and surgical intervention may be required later, but antibiotics should be administered as soon as possible. A tourniquet is not typically used in the management of open fractures unless there is life-threatening hemorrhage.

85. When treating a pregnant patient in cardiac arrest, which of the following interventions is most important for improving maternal and fetal outcomes?
a) Placing the patient in the left lateral position
b) Providing immediate cesarean section
c) Administering medications at lower doses
d) Avoiding chest compressions

Answer: a) Placing the patient in the left lateral position
Explanation: In a pregnant patient in cardiac arrest, placing the patient in the left lateral position is most important for improving maternal and fetal outcomes. This position helps to alleviate aortocaval compression and improves blood flow. Immediate cesarean section, adjusting medication doses, and avoiding chest compressions may be considered later in the management of the patient's condition.

86. When administering pain medication to a pediatric patient, which of the following considerations is most important?
a) Adjusting the dose based on the patient's weight
b) Choosing a medication with the least side effects
c) Using the same medication as for adults
d) Relying on parenteral administration

Answer: a) Adjusting the dose based on the patient's weight
Explanation: When administering pain medication to a pediatric patient, it is most important to adjust the dose based on the patient's weight. This ensures that the patient receives the appropriate amount of medication for their size. Choosing a medication with the least side effects, using the same medication as for adults, and relying on parenteral administration are secondary considerations.

87. A geriatric patient with a suspected hip fracture is being transported. What is the most appropriate method to minimize pain and discomfort during transport?
a) Applying a traction splint
b) Administering opioid analgesics
c) Immobilizing the limb with a vacuum splint
d) Encouraging the patient to ambulate

Answer: c) Immobilizing the limb with a vacuum splint

Explanation: Immobilizing the limb with a vacuum splint is the most appropriate method to minimize pain and discomfort during transport for geriatric patients with suspected hip fractures. Applying a traction splint or encouraging the patient to ambulate may exacerbate the injury, and administering opioid analgesics should be considered after immobilization.

88. Which of the following factors is most important to consider when treating a patient with a history of sickle cell disease who is experiencing severe pain?
a) Administering a blood transfusion
b) Encouraging the patient to drink fluids
c) Providing oxygen therapy
d) Initiating aggressive pain management

Answer: d) Initiating aggressive pain management

Explanation: Initiating aggressive pain management is the most important consideration when treating a patient with a history of sickle cell disease experiencing severe pain. Pain crises are common in sickle cell disease and require prompt pain control. Administering a blood transfusion, encouraging fluid intake, and providing oxygen therapy may be considered later in the management of the patient's condition.

89. In the context of cultural competence, which of the following is the most appropriate approach when interacting with a patient from a different cultural background?
a) Avoiding eye contact to show respect
b) Speaking slowly and loudly to ensure understanding
c) Adapting your communication style to the patient's preferences
d) Assuming the patient understands your instructions

Answer: c) Adapting your communication style to the patient's preferences

Explanation: Adapting your communication style to the patient's preferences is the most appropriate approach when interacting with a patient from a different cultural background. This shows respect and understanding for the patient's cultural norms and helps establish trust. Avoiding eye contact, speaking slowly and loudly, or assuming the patient understands your instructions may not be appropriate for all cultural backgrounds and may create misunderstandings.

90. When performing a pediatric assessment, which of the following components is unique to the pediatric primary survey?
a) Airway maintenance
b) Breathing and ventilation
c) Circulation with hemorrhage control
d) Disability and blood glucose check

Answer: d) Disability and blood glucose check

Explanation: In the pediatric primary survey, checking for disability and blood glucose is unique to pediatric patients. It is important to assess neurological status and blood glucose levels, as hypoglycemia may present with altered mental status in pediatric patients. Airway maintenance, breathing and ventilation, and circulation with hemorrhage control are components of both adult and pediatric primary surveys.

91. What is the most appropriate method for opening the airway in an unresponsive pediatric patient without a suspected cervical spine injury?
a) Jaw thrust maneuver
b) Head tilt-chin lift maneuver
c) Modified chin lift
d) Tongue-jaw lift

Answer: b) Head tilt-chin lift maneuver
Explanation: The head tilt-chin lift maneuver is the most appropriate method for opening the airway in an unresponsive pediatric patient without a suspected cervical spine injury. The jaw thrust maneuver is used when a cervical spine injury is suspected, while the modified chin lift and tongue-jaw lift are not standard techniques for pediatric airway management.

92. Which of the following pediatric patients is at the highest risk for developing hypothermia?
a) A child with a fever
b) A premature neonate
c) A child with bronchitis
d) A child with a sunburn

Answer: b) A premature neonate
Explanation: A premature neonate is at the highest risk for developing hypothermia due to their underdeveloped thermoregulation system and increased body surface area to volume ratio. Although fever, bronchitis, and sunburn may affect temperature regulation, these conditions do not pose as high a risk for hypothermia as prematurity.

93. In pediatric patients, which of the following factors is most likely to cause a decrease in cardiac output during a traumatic event?
a) Hypovolemia
b) Increased vascular resistance
c) Cardiogenic shock
d) Hypothermia

Answer: a) Hypovolemia
Explanation: In pediatric patients, hypovolemia is the most likely cause of decreased cardiac output during a traumatic event. Children have a limited ability to compensate for blood loss and are more susceptible to hypovolemic shock. Increased vascular resistance, cardiogenic shock, and hypothermia may also affect cardiac output but are less likely in pediatric trauma situations.

94. What is the most appropriate intervention for a pediatric patient experiencing a severe asthma attack?
a) Administer a short-acting beta-agonist
b) Initiate chest physiotherapy
c) Encourage slow, deep breaths
d) Provide supplemental oxygen only

Answer: a) Administer a short-acting beta-agonist

Explanation: Administering a short-acting beta-agonist, such as albuterol, is the most appropriate intervention for a pediatric patient experiencing a severe asthma attack. This medication helps to rapidly reverse bronchoconstriction and improve airflow. While chest physiotherapy, slow deep breaths, and supplemental oxygen may be helpful in some cases, they are not the primary intervention for severe asthma attacks.

95. Which of the following complications is most commonly associated with postpartum hemorrhage?
a) Uterine atony
b) Placenta previa
c) Placental abruption
d) Uterine rupture

Answer: a) Uterine atony

Explanation: Uterine atony, or the lack of uterine muscle contraction, is the most common cause of postpartum hemorrhage. Inadequate contraction of the uterus can lead to excessive bleeding following delivery. Placenta previa, placental abruption, and uterine rupture can also contribute to postpartum hemorrhage, but they are less common causes.

96. When assessing a pregnant patient with abdominal pain and vaginal bleeding, which of the following conditions should be considered?
a) Ectopic pregnancy
b) Gestational diabetes
c) Preeclampsia
d) Braxton-Hicks contractions

Answer: a) Ectopic pregnancy

Explanation: Ectopic pregnancy should be considered when assessing a pregnant patient presenting with abdominal pain and vaginal bleeding, as these are common symptoms of this potentially life-threatening condition. Gestational diabetes, preeclampsia, and Braxton-Hicks contractions do not typically present with these symptoms.

97. What is the most appropriate initial treatment for a pregnant patient experiencing a seizure due to eclampsia?
a) Administer magnesium sulfate
b) Perform immediate delivery
c) Begin anticonvulsant therapy
d) Administer high-flow oxygen

Answer: a) Administer magnesium sulfate

Explanation: The most appropriate initial treatment for a pregnant patient experiencing a seizure due to eclampsia is to administer magnesium sulfate, which can help prevent further seizures. While immediate delivery, anticonvulsant therapy, and high-flow oxygen may be necessary in some cases, the initial treatment should focus on seizure control with magnesium sulfate.

98. In a pregnant patient with a known history of placenta previa, which of the following signs and symptoms would be most concerning for an imminent delivery?
a) Contractions occurring every 10 minutes
b) Painless, bright red vaginal bleeding
c) Severe abdominal pain
d) Dark brown vaginal discharge

Answer: b) Painless, bright red vaginal bleeding
Explanation: Painless, bright red vaginal bleeding is the most concerning sign for an imminent delivery in a patient with a known history of placenta previa. This type of bleeding may indicate that the placenta is separating from the uterine wall, which can result in rapid blood loss and necessitate an emergency delivery. Contractions, severe abdominal pain, and dark brown vaginal discharge may be concerning in other situations, but they are less specific to placenta previa.

99. Which of the following maternal positions is most appropriate for managing a pregnant patient with a suspected cord prolapse during labor?
a) Supine
b) Lithotomy
c) Trendelenburg
d) Knee-chest

Answer: d) Knee-chest
Explanation: The knee-chest position is most appropriate for managing a pregnant patient with a suspected cord prolapse during labor. This position helps to relieve pressure on the umbilical cord, reducing the risk of fetal hypoxia. Supine, lithotomy, and Trendelenburg positions do not provide the same degree of pressure relief and are not as effective in managing cord prolapse.

100. Which of the following is the most appropriate initial intervention for a neonate with apnea and a heart rate below 60 beats per minute?
a) Positive pressure ventilation (PPV)
b) Chest compressions
c) Administration of epinephrine
d) Immediate intubation

Answer: a) Positive pressure ventilation (PPV)
Explanation: The most appropriate initial intervention for a neonate with apnea and a heart rate below 60 beats per minute is positive pressure ventilation (PPV). This helps to improve oxygenation and can increase the heart rate. If the heart rate remains below 60 beats per minute despite adequate ventilation, chest compressions should be initiated.

101. What is the recommended compression-to-ventilation ratio during neonatal CPR?
a) 15:2
b) 30:2
c) 3:1
d) 5:1

Answer: c) 3:1
Explanation: The recommended compression-to-ventilation ratio during neonatal CPR is 3:1. This means that for every three chest compressions, one breath should be given. This ratio provides adequate ventilation and perfusion for the neonate during resuscitation.

102. When should umbilical cord clamping be performed in a term neonate requiring resuscitation?
a) Immediately after birth
b) Within 30 seconds of birth
c) Within 60 seconds of birth
d) After the initiation of resuscitation

Answer: d) After the initiation of resuscitation
Explanation: In a term neonate requiring resuscitation, umbilical cord clamping should be performed after the initiation of resuscitation. This allows for the baby to receive some placental blood flow while resuscitation efforts are underway. For a baby not requiring resuscitation, delayed cord clamping (30-60 seconds) is recommended.

103. What is the most appropriate method for assessing the effectiveness of positive pressure ventilation during neonatal resuscitation?
a) Pulse oximetry
b) Chest rise
c) Heart rate
d) End-tidal carbon dioxide (ETCO2) monitoring

Answer: c) Heart rate
Explanation: The most appropriate method for assessing the effectiveness of positive pressure ventilation during neonatal resuscitation is monitoring the heart rate. An increasing heart rate is an indication of effective ventilation. While pulse oximetry, chest rise, and ETCO2 monitoring can provide additional information, heart rate is the most critical indicator of effective ventilation.

104. Which of the following conditions is most commonly associated with transient tachypnea of the newborn (TTN)?
a) Meconium aspiration syndrome
b) Respiratory distress syndrome
c) Persistent pulmonary hypertension
d) Delayed lung fluid clearance

Answer: d) Delayed lung fluid clearance
Explanation: Transient tachypnea of the newborn (TTN) is most commonly associated with delayed lung fluid clearance. This condition typically resolves within 24-72 hours after birth. Meconium aspiration syndrome, respiratory distress syndrome, and persistent pulmonary hypertension are all potential causes of respiratory distress in neonates but are not directly associated with TTN.

105. What is a common reason for geriatric patients to present with atypical signs and symptoms during an acute medical event?
a) Cognitive decline
b) Decreased pain perception
c) Increased medication use
d) Age-related physiological changes

Answer: d) Age-related physiological changes
Explanation: Age-related physiological changes can cause geriatric patients to present with atypical signs and symptoms during an acute medical event. These changes can affect the presentation of symptoms and make it more challenging to diagnose and manage their conditions.

106. Which of the following factors contributes most to the increased risk of medication-related complications in older adults?
a) Polypharmacy
b) Non-compliance with medication regimens
c) Reduced hepatic and renal function
d) Increased use of over-the-counter medications

Answer: c) Reduced hepatic and renal function
Explanation: Reduced hepatic and renal function in older adults contributes most to the increased risk of medication-related complications. As a result, older adults may have altered drug metabolism and excretion, increasing the risk of adverse drug reactions and interactions. Polypharmacy, non-compliance, and increased use of over-the-counter medications also contribute to the risk but are not the primary factors.

107. Which of the following conditions is a geriatric patient at higher risk for developing due to age-related changes in the immune system?
a) Osteoarthritis
b) Pneumonia
c) Hypertension
d) Diabetes mellitus

Answer: b) Pneumonia
Explanation: Due to age-related changes in the immune system, geriatric patients are at higher risk for developing pneumonia. These changes can lead to a decreased ability to fight infections, increasing their susceptibility to pneumonia and other infections.

108. In geriatric patients, which of the following assessment findings is more likely to be an indicator of an acute myocardial infarction (AMI)?
a) Sudden onset of severe chest pain
b) Shortness of breath and fatigue
c) Diaphoresis and nausea
d) Radiating pain to the left arm

Answer: b) Shortness of breath and fatigue
Explanation: In geriatric patients, an acute myocardial infarction (AMI) may present with atypical symptoms such as shortness of breath and fatigue, rather than the classic symptoms of chest pain and radiating pain. Geriatric patients may not experience the same level of pain due to age-related changes in pain perception.

109. When treating a geriatric patient with a suspected hip fracture, which of the following interventions is most appropriate for pain management?
a) Administering high-dose opioids
b) Applying ice to the affected area
c) Splinting the leg in a position of comfort
d) Administering nonsteroidal anti-inflammatory drugs (NSAIDs)

Answer: c) Splinting the leg in a position of comfort. Explanation: Splinting the leg in a position of comfort is the most appropriate intervention for pain management in a geriatric patient with a suspected hip fracture. This helps to minimize movement and provide support, reducing pain. Administering high-dose opioids may increase the risk of respiratory depression, while NSAIDs may not provide adequate pain relief and can have potential side effects. Applying ice is generally not recommended for hip fractures as it may not provide significant pain relief and can potentially cause harm.

110. During a mass casualty incident, what is the primary objective of triage?
a) To prioritize patients based on the severity of their injuries
b) To treat the most severely injured patients first
c) To transport all patients to the hospital as quickly as possible
d) To identify patients who can be treated on-scene and discharged

Answer: a) To prioritize patients based on the severity of their injuries. Explanation: The primary objective of triage during a mass casualty incident is to prioritize patients based on the severity of their injuries. This allows for the most efficient use of limited resources and ensures that those who are most critically injured receive care first.

111. What is the primary role of an incident commander during an emergency response operation?
a) To provide direct patient care
b) To establish and maintain command and control
c) To coordinate transportation of patients
d) To act as a liaison between responding agencies

Answer: b) To establish and maintain command and control. Explanation: The primary role of an incident commander during an emergency response operation is to establish and maintain command and control. This includes setting objectives, developing a response strategy, and coordinating resources to ensure a safe and effective response.

112. Which of the following best describes the role of a medical director in an emergency medical services (EMS) system?
a) To oversee daily operations and ensure adequate staffing
b) To provide medical oversight and establish treatment protocols
c) To coordinate with local hospitals and healthcare facilities
d) To supervise on-scene medical care during emergency incidents

Answer: b) To provide medical oversight and establish treatment protocols
Explanation: The role of a medical director in an EMS system is to provide medical oversight and establish treatment protocols. This includes developing and implementing clinical guidelines, ensuring quality assurance, and providing ongoing education and training for EMS personnel.

113. In a hazardous materials (HazMat) incident, what should EMS providers prioritize before attempting to provide patient care?
a) Identifying the specific hazardous material involved
b) Ensuring scene safety and donning appropriate personal protective equipment (PPE)
c) Initiating decontamination procedures for affected individuals
d) Notifying the appropriate authorities and requesting additional resources

Answer: b) Ensuring scene safety and donning appropriate personal protective equipment (PPE)
Explanation: Before attempting to provide patient care in a HazMat incident, EMS providers should prioritize ensuring scene safety and donning appropriate personal protective equipment (PPE). This helps to protect responders from potential harm and reduces the risk of cross-contamination.

114. Which of the following communication strategies is most effective when working with a language interpreter during a patient encounter?
a) Speak slowly and use simple language
b) Direct questions and statements to the interpreter
c) Use nonverbal cues and gestures to emphasize key points
d) Speak directly to the patient, maintaining eye contact

Answer: d) Speak directly to the patient, maintaining eye contact
Explanation: When working with a language interpreter during a patient encounter, it is most effective to speak directly to the patient while maintaining eye contact. This helps to establish rapport and ensure clear communication. The interpreter should be used as a conduit for communication, translating the message without becoming the focus of the conversation.

115. When providing a radio report to a receiving facility, which of the following components should be included in your patient presentation?
a) The patient's full name and home address
b) The patient's chief complaint, vital signs, and interventions performed
c) A detailed account of the patient's past medical history
d) The location where the patient was found and a description of the scene

Answer: b) The patient's chief complaint, vital signs, and interventions performed
Explanation: When providing a radio report to a receiving facility, it is important to include the patient's chief complaint, vital signs, and interventions performed. This information is crucial for the receiving facility to prepare for the patient's arrival and initiate appropriate care.

116. Which of the following is the most effective way to ensure clear communication when speaking with medical control over the radio?
a) Use plain language and avoid medical jargon
b) Use medical shorthand and abbreviations to save time
c) Speak quickly and loudly to ensure you are heard
d) Use a combination of medical terminology and plain language

Answer: a) Use plain language and avoid medical jargon. Explanation: Using plain language and avoiding medical jargon is the most effective way to ensure clear communication when speaking with medical control over the radio. This helps prevent misunderstandings and ensures that both parties understand the information being conveyed.

117. When communicating with a patient's family member, which of the following strategies is most appropriate for maintaining confidentiality?
a) Discussing the patient's condition in a public area to avoid making the family member uncomfortable
b) Providing only general information about the patient's condition and avoiding specific details
c) Sharing all relevant information about the patient's condition and treatment plan
d) Asking the family member to step away from the patient before discussing the patient's condition

Answer: b) Providing only general information about the patient's condition and avoiding specific details
Explanation: To maintain confidentiality when communicating with a patient's family member, it is best to provide only general information about the patient's condition and avoid specific details. This helps protect the patient's privacy while still keeping the family informed.

118. During a handoff report to the receiving facility, which of the following acronyms can be used to ensure a structured and thorough presentation?
a) SBAR (Situation, Background, Assessment, Recommendation)
b) SOAP (Subjective, Objective, Assessment, Plan)
c) SAMPLE (Symptoms, Allergies, Medications, Past medical history, Last oral intake, Events leading up to present illness)
d) OPQRST (Onset, Provocation, Quality, Radiation, Severity, Time)

Answer: a) SBAR (Situation, Background, Assessment, Recommendation). Explanation: The SBAR acronym (Situation, Background, Assessment, Recommendation) can be used during a handoff report to ensure a structured and thorough presentation. This method provides a clear and organized format for conveying essential patient information to the receiving facility.

119. How can you improve communication with a hearing-impaired patient during an emergency situation?
a) Speak louder and closer to the patient's ear
b) Use short, simple sentences and visual aids when possible
c) Rely primarily on nonverbal gestures to communicate
d) Ask the patient to read your lips while you speak

Answer: b) Use short, simple sentences and visual aids when possible. Explanation: To improve communication with a hearing-impaired patient during an emergency situation, use short, simple sentences and visual aids when possible. This can help facilitate understanding and ensure the patient receives appropriate care. It's also essential to be patient and allow the individual time to process the information being communicated.

120. During a mass casualty incident (MCI), which of the following triage systems is most commonly used to prioritize patients for treatment and transport?
a) START (Simple Triage and Rapid Treatment)
b) OPQRST (Onset, Provocation, Quality, Radiation, Severity, Time)
c) SAMPLE (Symptoms, Allergies, Medications, Past medical history, Last oral intake, Events leading up to present illness)
d) ABCDE (Airway, Breathing, Circulation, Disability, Exposure)

Answer: a) START (Simple Triage and Rapid Treatment)
Explanation: The START (Simple Triage and Rapid Treatment) system is most commonly used to prioritize patients during a mass casualty incident. This method allows for the rapid assessment and categorization of patients based on the severity of their injuries and their need for immediate medical attention.

121. When responding to a disaster, what is the primary goal of the Incident Command System (ICS)?
a) To ensure the safety of all responders and patients
b) To evacuate all non-essential personnel from the disaster area
c) To manage resources and coordinate the overall response effort
d) To provide medical care to the highest number of patients possible

Answer: c) To manage resources and coordinate the overall response effort
Explanation: The primary goal of the Incident Command System (ICS) when responding to a disaster is to manage resources and coordinate the overall response effort. This system is designed to provide a unified and organized approach to managing emergencies, ensuring that all responders work together effectively and efficiently.

122. In the context of disaster management, which of the following actions is considered a key principle of effective triage?
a) Treating the most severely injured patients first
b) Prioritizing patients based on their potential for survival
c) Providing immediate treatment to all patients in need
d) Transporting patients to the nearest hospital regardless of capacity

Answer: b) Prioritizing patients based on their potential for survival
Explanation: In disaster management, effective triage prioritizes patients based on their potential for survival. This approach ensures that limited resources are used to treat and transport those with the best chance of recovery, ultimately saving the greatest number of lives possible.

123. During a disaster response, which of the following is the most appropriate location for establishing a casualty collection point?
a) Close to the incident site, but in a safe and secure area
b) Inside a nearby building to provide shelter for patients
c) At the nearest hospital or medical facility
d) In a remote area, far away from the incident site

Answer: a) Close to the incident site, but in a safe and secure area
Explanation: During a disaster response, the most appropriate location for establishing a casualty collection point is close to the incident site, but in a safe and secure area. This allows for efficient triage, treatment, and transport of patients while minimizing the risk to both patients and responders.

124. What is the primary purpose of a disaster medical assistance team (DMAT)?
a) To provide immediate medical care in the aftermath of a disaster
b) To evacuate patients from the disaster area to a safe location
c) To provide logistical support and resource management during a disaster response
d) To coordinate the overall disaster response effort among various agencies

Answer: a) To provide immediate medical care in the aftermath of a disaster
Explanation: The primary purpose of a disaster medical assistance team (DMAT) is to provide immediate medical care in the aftermath of a disaster. These teams consist of medical professionals who are specially trained to respond to mass casualty incidents and can quickly deploy to provide medical support in the field.

125. What is the primary objective of quality improvement initiatives in emergency medical services (EMS)?
a) To increase revenue for EMS organizations
b) To reduce the workload of EMS personnel
c) To improve patient outcomes and enhance the quality of care
d) To minimize the number of calls to the EMS system

Answer: c) To improve patient outcomes and enhance the quality of care
Explanation: The primary objective of quality improvement initiatives in EMS is to improve patient outcomes and enhance the quality of care. These initiatives aim to identify and address areas of weakness, streamline processes, and implement best practices to ultimately provide better patient care.

126. Which of the following is a key component of a successful quality improvement program in EMS?
a) Punitive actions for errors and mistakes
b) Regular documentation audits
c) Continuous education and training
d) Strict adherence to protocols without flexibility

Answer: c) Continuous education and training
Explanation: Continuous education and training are key components of a successful quality improvement program in EMS. By providing ongoing learning opportunities, EMS personnel can stay up to date with best practices, refine their skills, and adapt to changes in protocols and guidelines, ultimately improving patient care.

127. In the context of EMS quality improvement, what is the purpose of a root cause analysis?
a) To determine which EMS provider is responsible for a patient's outcome
b) To identify the underlying cause of a problem or adverse event
c) To track the number of errors made during a specific time period
d) To establish new protocols and guidelines for patient care

Answer: b) To identify the underlying cause of a problem or adverse event

Explanation: In EMS quality improvement, the purpose of a root cause analysis is to identify the underlying cause of a problem or adverse event. By determining the root cause, EMS organizations can develop targeted interventions and strategies to prevent similar issues from occurring in the future, ultimately improving patient care.

128. Which of the following metrics is most relevant for measuring the effectiveness of an EMS quality improvement initiative?
a) Number of EMS calls per month
b) Average response time for EMS units
c) Patient satisfaction scores
d) Patient outcomes and clinical performance indicators

Answer: d) Patient outcomes and clinical performance indicators. Explanation: Patient outcomes and clinical performance indicators are the most relevant metrics for measuring the effectiveness of an EMS quality improvement initiative. These metrics help to assess the impact of quality improvement efforts on patient care, allowing organizations to identify areas where further improvement is needed.

129. How can EMS providers actively participate in quality improvement activities?
a) By refusing to follow new protocols and guidelines
b) By providing feedback and sharing experiences related to patient care
c) By focusing solely on their individual performance
d) By avoiding participation in quality improvement meetings

Answer: b) By providing feedback and sharing experiences related to patient care. Explanation: EMS providers can actively participate in quality improvement activities by providing feedback and sharing their experiences related to patient care. By openly discussing challenges, successes, and areas for improvement, EMS providers can contribute valuable insights and help shape the development and implementation of quality improvement initiatives.

130. Which of the following best describes the primary responsibility of a flight nurse during critical care transport?
a) Piloting the aircraft
b) Maintaining communication with air traffic control
c) Providing specialized care to critically ill or injured patients during transport
d) Coordinating ground transportation upon arrival at the destination

Answer: c) Providing specialized care to critically ill or injured patients during transport. Explanation: The primary responsibility of a flight nurse during critical care transport is to provide specialized care to critically ill or injured patients. Flight nurses are highly skilled professionals who are trained to manage complex medical situations during transport, ensuring the patient's safety and well-being.

131. Flight and transport nursing often involves which of the following types of patient transport?
a) Ground transport only
b) Air transport only
c) Both ground and air transport
d) Neither ground nor air transport

Answer: c) Both ground and air transport
Explanation: Flight and transport nursing can involve both ground and air transport, depending on the needs of the patient and the resources available. Flight nurses may work on fixed-wing aircraft, helicopters, or ground ambulances to provide critical care transport services.

132. In which of the following scenarios would a flight nurse be most likely to participate in the transport of a patient?
a) A stable patient requiring transport between hospitals for non-urgent diagnostic testing
b) A patient experiencing a life-threatening medical emergency in a remote area
c) A patient with minor injuries requiring transport to a nearby emergency department
d) A patient being discharged from the hospital to their home

Answer: b) A patient experiencing a life-threatening medical emergency in a remote area
Explanation: Flight nurses are most likely to participate in the transport of patients experiencing life-threatening medical emergencies, particularly in remote or hard-to-reach areas where rapid transport to a specialized medical facility is critical for the patient's survival and recovery.

133. Which of the following is an essential skill for a flight nurse to possess?
a) The ability to perform complex medical procedures in challenging environments
b) Expertise in aircraft maintenance and repair
c) Proficiency in speaking multiple languages
d) A background in aviation law and regulations

Answer: a) The ability to perform complex medical procedures in challenging environments
Explanation: Flight nurses must possess the ability to perform complex medical procedures in challenging environments. They are highly trained medical professionals who must be able to manage a wide range of medical conditions and emergencies while providing care during transport, often in confined spaces and under difficult conditions.

134. What is a key difference between the role of a flight nurse and that of a traditional nurse working in a hospital setting?
a) Flight nurses do not require any formal nursing education
b) Flight nurses have a more limited scope of practice than traditional nurses
c) Flight nurses work primarily in a transport setting, providing care to patients during critical care transport
d) Flight nurses do not collaborate with other healthcare professionals

Answer: c) Flight nurses work primarily in a transport setting, providing care to patients during critical care transport
Explanation: A key difference between the role of a flight nurse and that of a traditional nurse working in a hospital setting is that flight nurses work primarily in a transport setting, providing care to patients during critical care transport. While both roles require a strong foundation in nursing principles and practices, flight nurses must be able to adapt their skills to the unique challenges and constraints of the transport environment.

135. Which of the following advantages is associated with using a helicopter for patient transport in critical care situations?
a) Lower cost compared to other modes of transport
b) Ability to land directly at the scene of an incident
c) Longer range compared to fixed-wing aircraft
d) Larger capacity for patient and equipment

Answer: b) Ability to land directly at the scene of an incident
Explanation: One of the main advantages of using a helicopter for patient transport in critical care situations is its ability to land directly at the scene of an incident. This can be particularly beneficial in remote or hard-to-reach locations where rapid patient transport is crucial.

136. What is a primary disadvantage of using a fixed-wing aircraft for critical care transport?
a) Limited range
b) Need for a runway to take off and land
c) Inability to accommodate medical equipment
d) Slow speed compared to other modes of transport

Answer: b) Need for a runway to take off and land
Explanation: A primary disadvantage of using a fixed-wing aircraft for critical care transport is the need for a runway to take off and land. This can limit the accessibility of certain locations and may require additional ground transport to get the patient to and from the aircraft.

137. Which of the following is an advantage of using ground ambulances for patient transport in critical care situations?
a) Faster transport times compared to air transport
b) Lower risk of complications related to changes in altitude
c) Ability to bypass traffic and other obstacles on the road
d) More advanced medical equipment available on board

Answer: b) Lower risk of complications related to changes in altitude
Explanation: One advantage of using ground ambulances for patient transport in critical care situations is the lower risk of complications related to changes in altitude. Patients with certain medical conditions may be at increased risk for complications during air transport due to changes in air pressure and oxygen levels.

138. Which mode of transport is typically preferred for long-distance critical care transport when time is not a crucial factor?
a) Helicopter
b) Fixed-wing aircraft
c) Ground ambulance
d) All of the above

Answer: b) Fixed-wing aircraft
Explanation: Fixed-wing aircraft are typically preferred for long-distance critical care transport when time is not a crucial factor. Fixed-wing aircraft can cover greater distances and travel at faster speeds compared to helicopters and ground ambulances, making them a more efficient option for long-distance transport.

139. In which scenario would a ground ambulance be the most appropriate mode of transport for a critically ill patient?
a) The patient requires transport to a hospital 300 miles away
b) The patient is located in a remote area with no nearby road access
c) The patient needs to be transported a short distance between two hospitals within the same city
d) The patient needs to be airlifted from a disaster zone

Answer: c) The patient needs to be transported a short distance between two hospitals within the same city
Explanation: A ground ambulance would be the most appropriate mode of transport for a critically ill patient who needs to be transported a short distance between two hospitals within the same city. Ground ambulances can navigate urban environments effectively and are generally more cost-effective for short distances compared to air transport.

140. Which team member in a flight and transport nursing crew is primarily responsible for providing advanced medical care and interventions to the patient?
a) Pilot
b) Flight nurse
c) Paramedic
d) Respiratory therapist

Answer: b) Flight nurse
Explanation: The flight nurse is primarily responsible for providing advanced medical care and interventions to the patient during transport. Their role includes assessment, monitoring, and treatment of the patient's condition, as well as coordinating care with other team members.

141. In a typical flight and transport nursing crew configuration, who is responsible for operating the aircraft and ensuring safe navigation?
a) Flight nurse
b) Paramedic
c) Pilot
d) Respiratory therapist

Answer: c) Pilot
Explanation: The pilot is responsible for operating the aircraft and ensuring safe navigation during flight and transport nursing missions. Their primary focus is on the safe operation of the aircraft, while other team members attend to the medical needs of the patient.

142. Which crew member in a flight and transport nursing team may be responsible for managing a patient's airway and providing ventilator support?
a) Flight nurse
b) Paramedic
c) Pilot
d) Respiratory therapist

Answer: d) Respiratory therapist. Explanation: A respiratory therapist may be part of a flight and transport nursing team and is typically responsible for managing a patient's airway and providing ventilator support. They work closely with the flight nurse and other team members to ensure appropriate respiratory care is provided throughout the transport.

143. In some flight and transport nursing crew configurations, which team member may assist the flight nurse in providing medical care and interventions?
a) Pilot
b) Paramedic
c) Mechanic
d) Dispatcher

Answer: b) Paramedic. Explanation: In some crew configurations, a paramedic may be part of the team and assist the flight nurse in providing medical care and interventions. Paramedics have advanced training in emergency medical care and can support the flight nurse in managing the patient's condition during transport.

144. Which team member in a flight and transport nursing crew is responsible for coordinating communication between the transport team, medical control, and receiving facilities?
a) Pilot
b) Flight nurse
c) Paramedic
d) Communication specialist

Answer: d) Communication specialist. Explanation: A communication specialist may be part of a flight and transport nursing crew and is responsible for coordinating communication between the transport team, medical control, and receiving facilities. They facilitate the flow of information to ensure that all necessary parties are informed and updated about the patient's condition and transport status.

145. Crew resource management (CRM) is a critical aspect of safety and risk management in flight and transport nursing. What is the primary goal of CRM?
a) Increase efficiency in transport operations
b) Improve decision-making and communication among crew members
c) Decrease workload for individual crew members
d) Reduce the need for standardized protocols

Answer: b) Improve decision-making and communication among crew members. Explanation: The primary goal of CRM is to improve decision-making and communication among crew members. By fostering a culture of open communication and teamwork, CRM helps to ensure that all team members contribute to the safe and efficient management of the transport mission.

146. Which of the following risk mitigation strategies involves altering the mission or task to reduce the likelihood or severity of an adverse event?
a) Avoidance
b) Transference
c) Acceptance
d) Reduction

Answer: a) Avoidance
Explanation: Avoidance is a risk mitigation strategy that involves altering the mission or task to reduce the likelihood or severity of an adverse event. This may involve canceling or postponing a mission or changing the approach to a specific task based on risk assessment.

147. In flight and transport nursing, hazard identification is an essential part of safety and risk management. What is the primary purpose of hazard identification?
a) To assign blame for past incidents
b) To predict the likelihood of future incidents
c) To identify potential sources of harm and assess their risk
d) To develop new policies and procedures

Answer: c) To identify potential sources of harm and assess their risk
Explanation: The primary purpose of hazard identification is to identify potential sources of harm and assess their risk. By understanding the hazards present in the transport environment, teams can develop and implement strategies to manage and mitigate these risks, ultimately enhancing patient and crew safety.

148. Which of the following is NOT a principle of effective crew resource management in flight and transport nursing?
a) Open and honest communication
b) A strict hierarchy within the team
c) Shared decision-making
d) Mutual respect and trust

Answer: b) A strict hierarchy within the team
Explanation: Effective CRM encourages open and honest communication, shared decision-making, and mutual respect and trust among team members. A strict hierarchy within the team may impede open communication and collaboration, which are essential for effective CRM and overall safety and risk management.

149. In the context of safety and risk management in flight and transport nursing, what does the term "risk acceptance" refer to?
a) Ignoring identified risks and proceeding with a mission
b) Taking steps to reduce the likelihood or severity of an adverse event
c) Acknowledging and accepting a certain level of risk as part of the mission
d) Transferring the responsibility for managing risk to another party

Answer: c) Acknowledging and accepting a certain level of risk as part of the mission
Explanation: Risk acceptance refers to acknowledging and accepting a certain level of risk as part of the mission. In some cases, the potential benefits of a transport mission may outweigh the risks, and the team may decide to proceed with appropriate precautions and planning in place. Risk acceptance should be based on a thorough assessment and understanding of the risks involved.

150. Which of the following best describes the primary cause of hypoxia during flight?
a) Increased barometric pressure
b) Decreased barometric pressure
c) Increased oxygen concentration
d) Decreased oxygen concentration

Answer: b) Decreased barometric pressure
Explanation: Hypoxia is primarily caused by decreased barometric pressure during flight, which results in a lower partial pressure of oxygen in the inspired air. As altitude increases, the partial pressure of oxygen decreases, making it more difficult for the body to obtain adequate oxygen.

151. In aeromedical physiology, what is the primary concern related to decompression sickness?
a) The formation of gas bubbles in the blood and tissues
b) The expansion of trapped gases in body cavities
c) A rapid decrease in cabin pressure
d) The onset of hypoxia due to decreased barometric pressure

Answer: a) The formation of gas bubbles in the blood and tissues
Explanation: Decompression sickness is primarily caused by the formation of gas bubbles in the blood and tissues as a result of a rapid decrease in ambient pressure. These bubbles can cause pain, joint aches, neurological symptoms, and in severe cases, death.

152. Which of the following aircraft systems is responsible for maintaining cabin pressure during flight?
a) Environmental control system (ECS)
b) Electrical system
c) Fuel system
d) Hydraulic system

Answer: a) Environmental control system (ECS)
Explanation: The environmental control system (ECS) is responsible for maintaining cabin pressure during flight. It regulates airflow, temperature, and humidity within the aircraft cabin, ensuring a comfortable and safe environment for both patients and crew.

153. What is the primary reason for using supplemental oxygen during high-altitude flight?
a) To prevent the effects of hypoxia
b) To compensate for decreased cabin pressure
c) To increase the effectiveness of medical interventions
d) To prevent decompression sickness

Answer: a) To prevent the effects of hypoxia
Explanation: The primary reason for using supplemental oxygen during high-altitude flight is to prevent the effects of hypoxia. Supplemental oxygen helps maintain adequate oxygen saturation levels in the blood, ensuring the body's tissues receive sufficient oxygen to function properly.

154. Which of the following factors can exacerbate the effects of hypoxia in flight?
a) Low altitude
b) Increased oxygen concentration
c) High altitude
d) Adequate cabin pressure

Answer: c) High altitude
Explanation: High altitude can exacerbate the effects of hypoxia in flight. As altitude increases, barometric pressure decreases, which reduces the partial pressure of oxygen in the inspired air. This makes it more difficult for the body to obtain adequate oxygen, increasing the risk of hypoxia and its associated symptoms.

155. Which of the following is the most critical consideration for patient assessment in the flight and transport environment?
a) Patient privacy
b) Adequate lighting
c) Noise levels
d) Limited space

Answer: d) Limited space
Explanation: While all factors are important, limited space is the most critical consideration for patient assessment in the flight and transport environment. Space constraints can make it challenging to perform certain interventions or assessments, requiring flight nurses to adapt their approach and prioritize patient care based on available resources.

156. How can noise impact patient assessment during flight and transport?
a) It can cause communication challenges with the patient and other team members.
b) It can lead to increased patient anxiety.
c) It can impair the ability to auscultate breath sounds.
d) All of the above.

Answer: d) All of the above.
Explanation: Noise can impact patient assessment during flight and transport in several ways. It can cause communication challenges with the patient and other team members, lead to increased patient anxiety, and impair the ability to auscultate breath sounds, making it difficult to obtain accurate information about the patient's condition.

157. In the flight and transport environment, which triage category should be prioritized for transport?
a) Immediate
b) Delayed
c) Minimal
d) Expectant

Answer: a) Immediate
Explanation: Patients in the immediate triage category should be prioritized for transport in the flight and transport environment. These patients have life-threatening injuries or conditions that require immediate intervention and have the greatest chance of survival with timely care.

158. What is a key aspect of patient assessment that may be challenging in the flight and transport environment due to vibration?
a) Assessing skin color
b) Palpating for a pulse
c) Determining level of consciousness
d) Obtaining a medical history

Answer: b) Palpating for a pulse
Explanation: Palpating for a pulse may be challenging in the flight and transport environment due to vibration. The constant movement and vibrations from the aircraft or vehicle can make it difficult to accurately locate and assess a patient's pulse, potentially leading to inaccurate or incomplete assessment data.

159. When assessing a patient's respiratory status during transport, which of the following adaptations may be necessary due to the transport environment?
a) Using a stethoscope with noise-canceling capabilities
b) Relying solely on visual assessment
c) Increasing the oxygen flow rate
d) Assessing breath sounds at a higher frequency

Answer: a) Using a stethoscope with noise-canceling capabilities
Explanation: When assessing a patient's respiratory status during transport, using a stethoscope with noise-canceling capabilities may be necessary due to the transport environment. This allows for more accurate auscultation of breath sounds despite the high noise levels present during flight and ground transport.

160. Which of the following is a unique consideration for airway management during in-flight patient care?
a) Positioning the patient upright
b) Using an oropharyngeal airway
c) Limiting the use of sedatives
d) Considering the effects of altitude

Answer: d) Considering the effects of altitude
Explanation: During in-flight patient care, the effects of altitude on airway management must be considered. Changes in atmospheric pressure can lead to trapped gas expansion and increased airway resistance, which can affect the patient's respiratory status and the effectiveness of interventions.

161. What is the primary reason for providing oxygen therapy during in-flight patient care?
a) To prevent hypoxia
b) To decrease anxiety
c) To treat shock
d) To assist in pain management

Answer: a) To prevent hypoxia
Explanation: The primary reason for providing oxygen therapy during in-flight patient care is to prevent hypoxia. Due to the changes in atmospheric pressure during flight, the partial pressure of oxygen decreases, which can result in hypoxia if supplemental oxygen is not provided.

162. Which of the following ventilation strategies is most appropriate for managing a patient with respiratory distress during in-flight patient care?
a) Positive pressure ventilation
b) High-frequency oscillatory ventilation
c) Non-invasive positive pressure ventilation
d) Apneic oxygenation

Answer: c) Non-invasive positive pressure ventilation
Explanation: Non-invasive positive pressure ventilation (NIPPV) is the most appropriate ventilation strategy for managing a patient with respiratory distress during in-flight patient care. NIPPV can provide adequate ventilatory support without the need for invasive airway management, minimizing the risk of complications and allowing for easier care in the limited space of the transport environment.

163. How does the management of shock differ during in-flight patient care compared to ground-based care?
a) Fluid resuscitation should be more aggressive.
b) Vasopressor use should be minimized.
c) Fluid resuscitation should be more conservative.
d) Vasopressor use should be more aggressive.

Answer: c) Fluid resuscitation should be more conservative.
Explanation: Fluid resuscitation during in-flight patient care should be more conservative compared to ground-based care. The effects of altitude on intravascular volume and the potential for fluid shifts due to changes in cabin pressure may lead to fluid overload if aggressive fluid resuscitation is used.

164. In which critical condition is the administration of medications during in-flight patient care most likely to be affected by altitude-related changes?
a) Acute coronary syndrome
b) Seizures
c) Acute respiratory distress syndrome
d) Anaphylaxis

Answer: c) Acute respiratory distress syndrome
Explanation: In patients with acute respiratory distress syndrome (ARDS), the administration of medications during in-flight patient care may be affected by altitude-related changes. Changes in atmospheric pressure can affect drug absorption, distribution, metabolism, and excretion, which may require adjustments in medication dosing or administration. ARDS patients may be particularly sensitive to these changes due to the underlying respiratory pathology.

165. What is the primary purpose of using specialized transport ventilators during flight and transport nursing?
a) To minimize the size and weight of equipment
b) To provide advanced modes of ventilation
c) To account for changes in altitude and cabin pressure
d) To improve patient comfort during transport

Answer: c) To account for changes in altitude and cabin pressure
Explanation: Specialized transport ventilators are used during flight and transport nursing to account for changes in altitude and cabin pressure. These ventilators are designed to maintain consistent ventilation support despite the fluctuations in environmental conditions encountered during transport.

166. Which of the following monitoring tools is essential for flight and transport nursing due to its ability to continuously assess oxygenation levels?
a) End-tidal CO2 monitor
b) Pulse oximeter
c) Capnograph
d) Blood pressure monitor

Answer: b) Pulse oximeter
Explanation: A pulse oximeter is essential for flight and transport nursing because it continuously assesses oxygenation levels. This is crucial during transport, as changes in altitude can lead to hypoxia, making it important to monitor the patient's oxygen saturation closely.

167. What is the main advantage of using compact, multi-parameter monitors during flight and transport nursing?
a) They provide more accurate readings
b) They require less frequent calibration
c) They save space and weight in the transport environment
d) They are less expensive than traditional monitoring equipment

Answer: c) They save space and weight in the transport environment
Explanation: Compact, multi-parameter monitors are advantageous in flight and transport nursing because they save space and weight in the transport environment. This is important, as space and weight constraints are significant challenges during transport, and streamlined monitoring equipment can help optimize patient care.

168. Which specialized transport equipment is most appropriate for providing rapid, temporary circulatory support during flight and transport nursing?
a) Intra-aortic balloon pump (IABP)
b) Extracorporeal membrane oxygenation (ECMO)
c) Impella device
d) Ventricular assist device (VAD)

Answer: a) Intra-aortic balloon pump (IABP). Explanation: The intra-aortic balloon pump (IABP) is the most appropriate specialized transport equipment for providing rapid, temporary circulatory support during flight and transport nursing. IABPs are relatively portable and can be quickly implemented to support patients experiencing cardiogenic shock or other acute circulatory issues.

169. How does the use of transport isolette differ from a regular incubator during neonatal transport?
a) It provides a higher level of humidity
b) It has integrated monitoring capabilities
c) It is smaller and more portable
d) It offers additional thermal insulation

Answer: d) It offers additional thermal insulation

Explanation: Transport isolettes differ from regular incubators by offering additional thermal insulation. This is crucial during neonatal transport, as maintaining a stable, warm environment is critical for the well-being of the newborn, particularly in situations where the transport environment may be affected by fluctuations in temperature or cabin pressure.

170. What is the primary purpose of using the SBAR (Situation, Background, Assessment, Recommendation) communication tool during patient handoff in flight and transport nursing?
a) To provide a structured, concise format for relaying critical information
b) To assess the patient's overall status and condition
c) To establish rapport with the receiving healthcare team
d) To ensure that all required documentation is completed

Answer: a) To provide a structured, concise format for relaying critical information

Explanation: The primary purpose of using the SBAR communication tool during patient handoff is to provide a structured, concise format for relaying critical information. This helps ensure that important details are not missed and that the receiving healthcare team can quickly understand the patient's situation and needs.

171. Which of the following is an essential component of radio communication during flight and transport nursing?
a) Use of medical jargon to ensure accuracy
b) Speaking quickly to minimize radio transmission time
c) Maintaining patient confidentiality
d) Using the patient's full name to avoid confusion

Answer: c) Maintaining patient confidentiality

Explanation: Maintaining patient confidentiality is an essential component of radio communication during flight and transport nursing. This includes using patient identifiers that do not disclose personal information, such as age, gender, or medical record number, rather than using the patient's full name.

172. When documenting patient care during flight and transport nursing, which of the following should be prioritized?
a) Recording vital signs every 5 minutes
b) Documenting only significant interventions and assessments
c) Including as much detail as possible to create a comprehensive record
d) Focusing on the most critical interventions and assessments

Answer: d) Focusing on the most critical interventions and assessments

Explanation: When documenting patient care during flight and transport nursing, it is important to focus on the most critical interventions and assessments. This helps create a clear and concise record that can be easily reviewed by the receiving healthcare team and allows for efficient documentation during transport.

173. What is the primary goal of closed-loop communication in flight and transport nursing?
a) To ensure that all team members are aware of changes in patient status
b) To confirm that information has been received and understood
c) To facilitate open dialogue and feedback among team members
d) To encourage collaboration and decision-making within the team

Answer: b) To confirm that information has been received and understood
Explanation: The primary goal of closed-loop communication in flight and transport nursing is to confirm that information has been received and understood. This involves the sender providing information, the receiver repeating the information back to the sender, and the sender acknowledging that the receiver has understood the information correctly.

174. Why is it important to use plain language and avoid medical jargon when communicating with non-medical personnel during flight and transport nursing?
a) To save time and simplify communication
b) To ensure that everyone involved in the transport understands the situation
c) To minimize the risk of misinterpretation and errors
d) To maintain a professional and respectful tone

Answer: c) To minimize the risk of misinterpretation and errors
Explanation: It is important to use plain language and avoid medical jargon when communicating with non-medical personnel during flight and transport nursing to minimize the risk of misinterpretation and errors. This helps ensure that all parties involved in the transport have a clear understanding of the patient's needs and the care being provided.

175. Which of the following is the most appropriate approach for obtaining informed consent for a critical care transport?
a) Obtain verbal consent from the patient or their legal guardian
b) Have the patient sign a written consent form before transport
c) Assume consent based on the patient's medical condition and urgency of transport
d) Obtain consent from the patient's primary care physician

Answer: a) Obtain verbal consent from the patient or their legal guardian
Explanation: Informed consent is an essential component of the transport process. Ideally, verbal consent should be obtained from the patient or their legal guardian, as it is typically faster and more practical in emergency situations than written consent. However, in certain cases, implied consent may apply if the patient is unable to provide consent due to their medical condition.

176. Which of the following best describes the role of medical control in flight and transport nursing?
a) Providing real-time guidance on medical interventions during transport
b) Supervising and managing the transport team's performance
c) Ensuring that the transport is carried out safely and efficiently
d) Coordinating communication between the transport team and receiving facility

Answer: a) Providing real-time guidance on medical interventions during transport
Explanation: Medical control refers to the physician or medical professional who provides real-time guidance and authorization for medical interventions during transport. They help ensure that appropriate care is provided, taking into account the patient's condition, available resources, and the specific challenges of the transport environment.

177. Which of the following is an essential aspect of maintaining patient confidentiality during flight and transport nursing?
a) Sharing patient information only with members of the transport team
b) Using only the patient's initials when documenting their care
c) Limiting the discussion of patient information to secure communication channels
d) Ensuring that the patient's medical record number is not disclosed

Answer: c) Limiting the discussion of patient information to secure communication channels
Explanation: Maintaining patient confidentiality during flight and transport nursing involves limiting the discussion of patient information to secure communication channels, such as encrypted radios or secure messaging apps. This helps protect sensitive information from being intercepted or overheard by unauthorized individuals.

178. When a flight nurse encounters an ethical dilemma during transport, which of the following should be the primary guiding principle?
a) The flight nurse's personal beliefs and values
b) The patient's wishes and preferences
c) The policies and protocols of the transport service
d) The best interests of the patient

Answer: d) The best interests of the patient
Explanation: When faced with an ethical dilemma during transport, the primary guiding principle should be the best interests of the patient. This involves considering the patient's wishes and preferences, as well as the medical and ethical standards of care, to make decisions that prioritize the patient's well-being and autonomy.

179. In the context of flight and transport nursing, which of the following statements best describes the concept of autonomy?
a) The right of patients to make informed decisions about their care
b) The ability of flight nurses to practice independently of medical control
c) The freedom of transport services to establish their own policies and procedures
d) The responsibility of flight nurses to advocate for the needs of their patients

Answer: a) The right of patients to make informed decisions about their care
Explanation: Autonomy, in the context of flight and transport nursing, refers to the right of patients to make informed decisions about their care. This includes the right to consent to or refuse treatment, as well as the right to be informed about the risks and benefits of proposed interventions. Respecting patient autonomy is an essential aspect of ethical care in the transport environment.

180. Which of the following best describes the relationship between altitude and the partial pressure of oxygen (PO2) during air transport?
a) PO2 remains constant regardless of altitude
b) PO2 increases as altitude increases
c) PO2 decreases as altitude increases
d) PO2 fluctuates depending on cabin pressure

Answer: c) PO2 decreases as altitude increases

Explanation: As altitude increases, the partial pressure of oxygen (PO2) decreases. This can lead to a decrease in the patient's blood oxygen levels, which may exacerbate underlying medical conditions or lead to hypoxia if not appropriately managed.

181. Which of the following is a potential consequence of the decreased atmospheric pressure experienced during air transport?
a) Increased blood viscosity
b) Expansion of trapped gases
c) Decreased cardiac output
d) Vasoconstriction

Answer: b) Expansion of trapped gases

Explanation: Decreased atmospheric pressure during air transport can cause trapped gases to expand. This may lead to complications such as increased intracranial pressure, worsening pneumothorax, or abdominal distention in patients with gastrointestinal air.

182. In order to prevent hypoxia during air transport, which of the following strategies is most appropriate?
a) Administer oxygen therapy as needed based on pulse oximetry readings
b) Increase cabin pressure to sea level
c) Provide supplemental oxygen to all patients regardless of their condition
d) Limit the altitude of the transport aircraft

Answer: a) Administer oxygen therapy as needed based on pulse oximetry readings

Explanation: To prevent hypoxia during air transport, it is essential to closely monitor patients' oxygenation status and administer oxygen therapy as needed based on pulse oximetry readings. This approach allows for individualized care and ensures that patients receive the appropriate level of oxygen support.

183. How can flight nurses manage the impact of temperature fluctuations during air transport?
a) Adjust the aircraft's heating and cooling systems as needed
b) Use passive warming or cooling measures, such as blankets and ice packs
c) Administer medications to regulate the patient's body temperature
d) Both a) and b)

Answer: d) Both a) and b)

Explanation: To manage temperature fluctuations during air transport, flight nurses can adjust the aircraft's heating and cooling systems as needed and use passive warming or cooling measures, such as blankets and ice packs. These strategies can help maintain a comfortable and stable environment for the patient and minimize the risk of temperature-related complications.

184. What is the primary reason for considering cabin pressure changes when administering intravenous (IV) medications during air transport?
a) Changes in cabin pressure can affect the rate of drug absorption
b) Changes in cabin pressure can cause air bubbles in the IV line
c) Changes in cabin pressure can alter the potency of the medication
d) Changes in cabin pressure can affect the patient's level of consciousness

Answer: a) Changes in cabin pressure can affect the rate of drug absorption
Explanation: Cabin pressure changes during air transport can affect the rate of drug absorption for intravenous (IV) medications. Flight nurses should be aware of this potential impact and adjust the administration rate accordingly to ensure that the patient receives the appropriate dose and therapeutic effect.

185. Which of the following is a primary goal of effective communication among crew members, the dispatch center, and receiving facilities during patient transport?
a) Minimizing the need for decision-making during transport
b) Ensuring a smooth and coordinated patient care process
c) Reducing the amount of time spent in the transport vehicle
d) Demonstrating professionalism and competence to the patient

Answer: b) Ensuring a smooth and coordinated patient care process
Explanation: Effective communication among all parties involved in patient transport is crucial for ensuring a smooth and coordinated patient care process. Clear and timely communication helps prevent misunderstandings, reduce errors, and promote efficient patient care.

186. What communication technique is most useful for overcoming the impact of noise and distractions during patient transport?
a) Raising your voice to ensure others can hear you
b) Repeating critical information to confirm understanding
c) Using non-verbal communication, such as hand signals
d) Using electronic messaging to relay information

Answer: b) Repeating critical information to confirm understanding
Explanation: Repeating critical information and using closed-loop communication can help overcome the impact of noise and distractions during patient transport. This technique ensures that all parties have heard and understood the information, minimizing the risk of miscommunication.

187. How can transport nurses overcome communication barriers related to language differences between the transport team and receiving facility staff?
a) Use a translation app or device to facilitate communication
b) Speak more slowly and use simple language
c) Rely on non-verbal communication, such as gestures
d) Coordinate with an interpreter, either in person or remotely

Answer: d) Coordinate with an interpreter, either in person or remotely
Explanation: When language differences are a barrier to effective communication, coordinating with an interpreter, either in person or remotely, can help facilitate clear and accurate communication between the transport team and receiving facility staff.

188. What is the primary purpose of using a standardized handoff report during patient transport?
a) To ensure all relevant patient information is communicated to the receiving facility
b) To minimize the time spent discussing the patient's condition
c) To establish the transport nurse's authority and expertise
d) To ensure compliance with legal and regulatory requirements

Answer: a) To ensure all relevant patient information is communicated to the receiving facility

Explanation: The primary purpose of using a standardized handoff report during patient transport is to ensure that all relevant patient information is communicated to the receiving facility staff. This helps promote continuity of care and reduces the risk of errors or omissions in the patient's treatment.

189. Which of the following strategies can help improve communication and coordination among transport nursing crew members during patient transport?
a) Use a designated team leader to direct communication and decision-making
b) Limit communication to only essential information to minimize distractions
c) Assign specific roles and responsibilities to each crew member
d) Both a) and c)

Answer: d) Both a) and c)

Explanation: Designating a team leader to direct communication and decision-making, as well as assigning specific roles and responsibilities to each crew member, can help improve communication and coordination during patient transport. This approach helps to establish clear lines of communication, streamline decision-making, and promote efficient patient care.

190. What is the primary purpose of a pre-flight safety briefing in flight and ground transport?
a) To assess the patient's understanding of their condition
b) To identify potential hazards and review safety protocols
c) To ensure that all crew members are familiar with the patient's medical history
d) To review the transport route and expected weather conditions

Answer: b) To identify potential hazards and review safety protocols

Explanation: The primary purpose of a pre-flight safety briefing is to identify potential hazards and review safety protocols with the transport team. This process helps ensure that all crew members are aware of potential risks and understand their responsibilities in maintaining a safe transport environment.

191. Which of the following is an essential piece of safety equipment that should be available during flight and ground transport?
a) A portable GPS device for navigation
b) Personal protective equipment (PPE) for crew members
c) Noise-canceling headphones for the patient
d) An automated external defibrillator (AED)

Answer: d) An automated external defibrillator (AED)

Explanation: An AED is an essential piece of safety equipment that should be available during flight and ground transport. It can be used to deliver a potentially lifesaving shock to a patient experiencing sudden cardiac arrest, which can occur unexpectedly during transport.

192. How can transport nurses contribute to maintaining a safe environment during patient transport?
a) Regularly inspecting and maintaining transport equipment
b) Monitoring the patient's condition and responding to changes appropriately
c) Ensuring all crew members are well-rested and alert
d) All of the above

Answer: d) All of the above
Explanation: Transport nurses play a critical role in maintaining a safe transport environment by regularly inspecting and maintaining transport equipment, monitoring the patient's condition and responding to changes appropriately, and ensuring that all crew members are well-rested and alert.

193. What is the primary goal of crew resource management (CRM) in flight and ground transport?
a) To reduce crew workload and improve efficiency
b) To enhance communication and teamwork among crew members
c) To ensure that the transport team adheres to standard operating procedures
d) To provide a structured approach to training and professional development

Answer: b) To enhance communication and teamwork among crew members
Explanation: Crew resource management (CRM) is a system designed to enhance communication and teamwork among crew members during flight and ground transport. By improving communication, decision-making, and problem-solving skills, CRM aims to reduce the risk of errors and enhance patient safety.

194. Which of the following strategies can help minimize the risk of patient injury during transport, particularly during takeoff, landing, and ground ambulance movement?
a) Ensuring the patient is securely fastened to the transport stretcher
b) Administering sedatives or analgesics to reduce patient discomfort
c) Placing padding around the patient's extremities
d) Adjusting the transport vehicle's suspension system to minimize vibration

Answer: a) Ensuring the patient is securely fastened to the transport stretcher
Explanation: Ensuring the patient is securely fastened to the transport stretcher can help minimize the risk of patient injury during transport, particularly during takeoff, landing, and ground ambulance movement. Proper patient restraint helps to prevent movement-related injuries and maintain the patient's position during transport.

195. A patient develops sudden chest pain, shortness of breath, and tachycardia during air transport. Which of the following should be considered as a possible cause?
a) Acute myocardial infarction
b) Pulmonary embolism
c) Tension pneumothorax
d) All of the above

Answer: d) All of the above
Explanation: All of the conditions listed could cause sudden chest pain, shortness of breath, and tachycardia during air transport. The flight nurse should perform a thorough assessment and initiate appropriate interventions based on the patient's clinical presentation.

196. A patient experiencing an anaphylactic reaction during air transport requires immediate intervention. What is the first-line medication for anaphylaxis?
a) Epinephrine
b) Diphenhydramine
c) Albuterol
d) Methylprednisolone

Answer: a) Epinephrine. Explanation: Epinephrine is the first-line medication for anaphylaxis. It should be administered promptly to counteract the life-threatening symptoms of anaphylaxis, such as airway constriction, hypotension, and shock.

197. During air transport, a patient with a history of seizures experiences a generalized tonic-clonic seizure. What is the most appropriate initial intervention?
a) Administering a benzodiazepine, such as lorazepam or diazepam
b) Restraining the patient to prevent injury
c) Placing the patient in a supine position to facilitate breathing
d) Starting an intravenous antiepileptic medication

Answer: a) Administering a benzodiazepine, such as lorazepam or diazepam. Explanation: The most appropriate initial intervention for a patient experiencing a generalized tonic-clonic seizure during air transport is administering a benzodiazepine, such as lorazepam or diazepam. This medication can help to stop the seizure and reduce the risk of further complications.

198. A patient with a history of congestive heart failure develops acute respiratory distress during flight. Which of the following interventions is most appropriate for this situation?
a) Administering high-flow oxygen
b) Initiating noninvasive positive pressure ventilation (NIPPV)
c) Administering a loop diuretic, such as furosemide
d) Performing endotracheal intubation and mechanical ventilation

Answer: b) Initiating noninvasive positive pressure ventilation (NIPPV). Explanation: Initiating noninvasive positive pressure ventilation (NIPPV) is the most appropriate intervention for a patient with acute respiratory distress related to congestive heart failure. NIPPV can help to improve oxygenation, reduce the work of breathing, and decrease the need for intubation and mechanical ventilation.

199. A patient with a history of hypertension develops a severe headache and altered mental status during flight. What is the most likely cause, and what should be the primary intervention?
a) Migraine; administer a triptan medication
b) Hypoglycemia; administer oral glucose or intravenous dextrose
c) Hypertensive emergency; administer an antihypertensive medication
d) Stroke; administer tissue plasminogen activator (tPA)

Answer: c) Hypertensive emergency; administer an antihypertensive medication. Explanation: A severe headache and altered mental status in a patient with a history of hypertension during flight may indicate a hypertensive emergency. The primary intervention should be administering an antihypertensive medication to lower the patient's blood pressure and reduce the risk of end-organ damage.

200. Which of the following transport ventilators is best suited for managing patients with severe acute respiratory distress syndrome (ARDS)?
a) Volume-cycled ventilator
b) Pressure-cycled ventilator
c) Transport ventilator with pressure control and inverse ratio ventilation (IRV) capabilities
d) Basic bag-valve-mask device

Answer: c) Transport ventilator with pressure control and inverse ratio ventilation (IRV) capabilities
Explanation: A transport ventilator with pressure control and inverse ratio ventilation (IRV) capabilities is best suited for managing patients with severe ARDS. This type of ventilator can provide more precise control over airway pressures and ventilation times, which can help minimize lung injury and improve gas exchange in patients with ARDS.

201. During patient transport, which of the following monitoring tools is most useful for detecting and managing potential complications related to central venous catheters?
a) End-tidal CO2 monitor
b) Pulse oximeter
c) Invasive blood pressure monitor
d) Ultrasound machine

Answer: d) Ultrasound machine
Explanation: An ultrasound machine is most useful for detecting and managing potential complications related to central venous catheters during patient transport. Ultrasound can help visualize the position of the catheter, assess for complications such as pneumothorax or vascular injury, and guide any necessary interventions.

202. A transport nurse is preparing to initiate a continuous intravenous infusion of a vasopressor medication for a critically ill patient. Which of the following infusion devices would be most appropriate for this purpose?
a) Syringe pump
b) Volumetric infusion pump
c) Gravity drip infusion set
d) Elastomeric infusion device

Answer: a) Syringe pump
Explanation: A syringe pump is the most appropriate infusion device for initiating a continuous intravenous infusion of a vasopressor medication in a critically ill patient. Syringe pumps provide precise control over infusion rates and are well-suited for administering small volumes of high-risk medications, such as vasopressors.

203. In addition to standard vital sign monitoring, which of the following is a crucial monitoring parameter for a patient on mechanical ventilation during transport?
a) Central venous pressure
b) End-tidal CO2
c) Intra-abdominal pressure
d) Serum lactate level

Answer: b) End-tidal CO2
Explanation: End-tidal CO2 monitoring is crucial for patients on mechanical ventilation during transport. It provides continuous, noninvasive assessment of ventilation and can help detect changes in the patient's respiratory status, such as airway obstruction, hypoventilation, or dislodged endotracheal tube.

204. Regular equipment maintenance is essential for ensuring the safe operation of transport equipment. Which of the following is a key component of proper equipment maintenance?
a) Conducting a visual inspection of all equipment before each transport
b) Performing regular equipment calibration
c) Replacing equipment according to the manufacturer's recommended schedule
d) All of the above

Answer: d) All of the above
Explanation: Proper equipment maintenance includes conducting a visual inspection of all equipment before each transport, performing regular equipment calibration, and replacing equipment according to the manufacturer's recommended schedule. These steps help to ensure the safe operation of transport equipment and minimize the risk of equipment-related complications during patient transport.

205. Which of the following is NOT a common sign of respiratory distress in a patient during transport?
a) Tachypnea
b) Use of accessory muscles
c) Cyanosis
d) Bradycardia

Answer: d) Bradycardia. Explanation: Bradycardia is not a common sign of respiratory distress. Tachypnea, use of accessory muscles, and cyanosis are all signs of respiratory distress. Patients in respiratory distress typically have an increased heart rate (tachycardia) rather than a decreased heart rate (bradycardia).

206. Early recognition of respiratory distress is essential for preventing complications during transport. Which of the following assessment techniques is LEAST helpful in identifying respiratory distress?
a) Observing the patient's breathing pattern
b) Palpating the chest for crepitus
c) Listening to lung sounds with a stethoscope
d) Measuring oxygen saturation with a pulse oximeter

Answer: b) Palpating the chest for crepitus. Explanation: While palpating the chest for crepitus can provide valuable information about the presence of subcutaneous emphysema or rib fractures, it is not the most helpful assessment technique for identifying respiratory distress. Observing the patient's breathing pattern, listening to lung sounds, and measuring oxygen saturation are more directly related to identifying respiratory distress.

207. What is the first step in managing a patient experiencing respiratory distress during transport?
a) Administering supplemental oxygen
b) Initiating noninvasive ventilation
c) Ensuring a patent airway
d) Preparing for intubation

Answer: c) Ensuring a patent airway. Explanation: The first step in managing a patient experiencing respiratory distress during transport is ensuring a patent airway. A clear airway is essential for effective oxygenation and ventilation. Once the airway is secured, other interventions such as supplemental oxygen, noninvasive ventilation, or intubation may be considered based on the patient's needs.

208. A patient experiencing respiratory distress during transport has an oxygen saturation of 89% on room air. Which of the following interventions is most appropriate for this patient?
a) Administering a bronchodilator
b) Initiating noninvasive positive pressure ventilation (NIPPV)
c) Administering supplemental oxygen
d) Rapid sequence intubation

Answer: c) Administering supplemental oxygen. Explanation: Administering supplemental oxygen is the most appropriate intervention for a patient with an oxygen saturation of 89% on room air. Supplemental oxygen can help improve oxygenation and alleviate respiratory distress. Other interventions, such as bronchodilators, NIPPV, or intubation, may be considered based on the patient's underlying condition and response to initial therapy.

209. Which of the following patients would be MOST likely to benefit from noninvasive positive pressure ventilation (NIPPV) during transport?
a) A patient with severe asthma exacerbation and impending respiratory failure
b) A patient with a suspected tension pneumothorax
c) A patient with acute pulmonary edema due to congestive heart failure
d) A patient with severe facial trauma and airway obstruction

Answer: c) A patient with acute pulmonary edema due to congestive heart failure
Explanation: A patient with acute pulmonary edema due to congestive heart failure is most likely to benefit from NIPPV during transport. NIPPV can help to improve oxygenation and decrease the work of breathing in patients with acute pulmonary edema. In contrast, NIPPV may not be appropriate or effective for patients with severe asthma exacerbation, tension pneumothorax, or airway obstruction due to facial trauma.

210. Which of the following is NOT a common cause of airway obstruction in a patient during transport?
a) Foreign body aspiration
b) Tongue falling back into the throat
c) Epiglottitis
d) Hyperventilation

Answer: d) Hyperventilation. Explanation: Hyperventilation is not a common cause of airway obstruction. Foreign body aspiration, tongue falling back into the throat, and epiglottitis are all potential causes of airway obstruction during transport.

211. A patient with an obstructed airway may present with which of the following clinical signs?
a) Stridor
b) Wheezing
c) Crackles
d) Diminished breath sounds

Answer: a) Stridor
Explanation: Stridor is a high-pitched, harsh sound that can be heard during inspiration or expiration and is indicative of upper airway obstruction. Wheezing, crackles, and diminished breath sounds are more commonly associated with lower airway or lung issues.

212. What is the most critical intervention for managing a patient with a complete airway obstruction during transport?
a) Administration of a bronchodilator
b) Manual removal of the foreign body
c) Rapid sequence intubation
d) Needle cricothyroidotomy

Answer: b) Manual removal of the foreign body
Explanation: In cases of complete airway obstruction, the most critical intervention is to remove the foreign body, often using techniques like back blows, chest thrusts, or finger sweeps. Other interventions, such as bronchodilators, intubation, or needle cricothyroidotomy, may be considered if appropriate but are not the primary interventions for a complete airway obstruction.

213. Which of the following interventions is generally NOT appropriate for managing partial airway obstruction in a conscious patient during transport?
a) Encouraging the patient to cough forcefully
b) Performing the Heimlich maneuver
c) Administration of oxygen
d) Monitoring the patient's airway and breathing

Answer: b) Performing the Heimlich maneuver
Explanation: The Heimlich maneuver should not be used for conscious patients with partial airway obstruction, as it may inadvertently cause a complete obstruction. Encouraging the patient to cough, administering oxygen, and monitoring the patient's airway and breathing are appropriate interventions for a conscious patient with a partial airway obstruction.

214. Which of the following airway management techniques is most appropriate for a patient with severe facial trauma and airway obstruction during transport?
a) Orotracheal intubation
b) Nasotracheal intubation
c) Needle cricothyroidotomy
d) Bag-valve-mask ventilation

Answer: c) Needle cricothyroidotomy
Explanation: Needle cricothyroidotomy is the most appropriate airway management technique for a patient with severe facial trauma and airway obstruction, as it bypasses the upper airway and establishes a temporary airway. Orotracheal intubation, nasotracheal intubation, and bag-valve-mask ventilation may not be feasible or effective in patients with severe facial trauma and airway obstruction.

215. What is the primary goal of mechanical ventilation during patient transport?
a) To provide adequate oxygenation
b) To minimize work of breathing
c) To maintain appropriate lung volumes
d) All of the above

Answer: d) All of the above

Explanation: The primary goal of mechanical ventilation during patient transport is to provide adequate oxygenation, minimize the work of breathing, and maintain appropriate lung volumes to ensure optimal patient care.

216. Which of the following modes of mechanical ventilation allows the patient to initiate their own breaths while the ventilator delivers a set tidal volume?
a) Assist-control ventilation (ACV)
b) Synchronized intermittent mandatory ventilation (SIMV)
c) Pressure support ventilation (PSV)
d) Continuous positive airway pressure (CPAP)

Answer: b) Synchronized intermittent mandatory ventilation (SIMV). Explanation: SIMV allows the patient to initiate their own breaths while the ventilator delivers a set tidal volume. ACV delivers a set tidal volume for every breath, regardless of whether the patient initiates the breath or the ventilator does. PSV and CPAP provide pressure support for spontaneous breaths but do not deliver a set tidal volume.

217. What is the most crucial parameter to monitor and adjust when managing a patient on a mechanical ventilator during transport?
a) Tidal volume
b) Respiratory rate
c) Oxygen saturation
d) Inspiratory time

Answer: c) Oxygen saturation. Explanation: Oxygen saturation is the most crucial parameter to monitor and adjust during transport, as it is an indirect measure of the patient's oxygenation. While tidal volume, respiratory rate, and inspiratory time are essential parameters to consider, they are not as directly indicative of the patient's oxygenation status.

218. Which of the following ventilator settings is typically adjusted to manage a patient's carbon dioxide levels during transport?
a) FiO2
b) PEEP
c) Inspiratory time
d) Respiratory rate

Answer: d) Respiratory rate. Explanation: Respiratory rate is typically adjusted to manage a patient's carbon dioxide levels during transport. Increasing the respiratory rate can help eliminate more carbon dioxide, while decreasing the respiratory rate can retain more carbon dioxide. FiO2, PEEP, and inspiratory time are more focused on managing oxygenation and lung volumes.

219. When managing a patient on mechanical ventilation during transport, which of the following is an essential safety measure?
a) Preoxygenating the patient before transport
b) Having a backup ventilation device available
c) Administering a sedative to the patient
d) Using a transport ventilator with a heated humidifier

Answer: b) Having a backup ventilation device available
Explanation: Having a backup ventilation device, such as a bag-valve-mask, available is an essential safety measure during transport, as it ensures that the patient can be ventilated manually in case of ventilator failure or other issues. Preoxygenating the patient, administering a sedative, and using a heated humidifier are all helpful in specific situations but are not as universally important for ensuring patient safety during transport.

220. Which of the following is a common cause of acute respiratory failure?
a) Pulmonary embolism
b) Heart failure
c) Pneumonia
d) All of the above

Answer: d) All of the above
Explanation: Acute respiratory failure can be caused by various factors, including pulmonary embolism, heart failure, and pneumonia. It is crucial to identify the underlying cause to guide appropriate management strategies during transport.

221. In the context of acute respiratory failure, what is the primary goal of supplemental oxygen therapy?
a) Increase the patient's oxygen saturation
b) Decrease the patient's work of breathing
c) Improve ventilation-perfusion mismatch
d) Prevent the need for mechanical ventilation

Answer: a) Increase the patient's oxygen saturation
Explanation: The primary goal of supplemental oxygen therapy in acute respiratory failure is to increase the patient's oxygen saturation, ensuring adequate oxygen delivery to tissues. While supplemental oxygen may help decrease the work of breathing, improve ventilation-perfusion mismatch, and prevent the need for mechanical ventilation, these are secondary goals.

222. Which non-invasive ventilation method is commonly used to manage patients with acute respiratory failure due to cardiogenic pulmonary edema?
a) Continuous positive airway pressure (CPAP)
b) Bilevel positive airway pressure (BiPAP)
c) High-flow nasal cannula (HFNC)
d) Nasal mask ventilation

Answer: a) Continuous positive airway pressure (CPAP)
Explanation: CPAP is commonly used to manage patients with acute respiratory failure due to cardiogenic pulmonary edema, as it helps to improve oxygenation and reduce preload and afterload. BiPAP, HFNC, and nasal mask ventilation can also be used in certain situations, but CPAP is generally considered the first-line therapy for cardiogenic pulmonary edema.

223. In a patient with acute respiratory failure who is unresponsive to non-invasive ventilation, what is the next step in management?
a) Increase supplemental oxygen flow rate
b) Administer bronchodilators
c) Initiate invasive mechanical ventilation
d) Administer diuretics

Answer: c) Initiate invasive mechanical ventilation
Explanation: If a patient with acute respiratory failure is unresponsive to non-invasive ventilation, the next step is typically to initiate invasive mechanical ventilation. This provides better control over the patient's oxygenation and ventilation, ensuring adequate gas exchange. While increasing supplemental oxygen, administering bronchodilators, or giving diuretics may be helpful in some cases, these interventions are generally not sufficient for managing severe respiratory failure.

224. What is a potential complication of invasive mechanical ventilation in patients with acute respiratory failure?
a) Barotrauma
b) Oxygen toxicity
c) Aspiration
d) All of the above

Answer: d) All of the above
Explanation: Invasive mechanical ventilation can cause various complications, including barotrauma, oxygen toxicity, and aspiration. It is essential to monitor patients closely during transport and adjust ventilator settings as needed to minimize the risk of these complications.

225. What is the primary pharmacologic treatment for an asthma exacerbation during transport?
a) Inhaled short-acting beta-agonists (SABAs)
b) Intravenous corticosteroids
c) Inhaled anticholinergics
d) Intravenous magnesium sulfate

Answer: a) Inhaled short-acting beta-agonists (SABAs)
Explanation: The primary pharmacologic treatment for an asthma exacerbation during transport is inhaled short-acting beta-agonists, such as albuterol. They provide rapid bronchodilation, which helps improve airflow and relieve symptoms. Other treatments, such as intravenous corticosteroids, inhaled anticholinergics, and intravenous magnesium sulfate, may be used as adjunct therapies depending on the severity of the exacerbation.

226. Which of the following signs might indicate a COPD exacerbation during transport?
a) Increased wheezing
b) Change in sputum color or quantity
c) Increased shortness of breath
d) All of the above

Answer: d) All of the above
Explanation: A COPD exacerbation may present with increased wheezing, a change in sputum color or quantity, and increased shortness of breath. During transport, it is crucial to monitor the patient closely for any signs of exacerbation and initiate appropriate interventions as needed.

227. What is the primary cause of cardiogenic pulmonary edema?
a) Fluid overload
b) Left ventricular failure
c) Pneumonia
d) Chronic obstructive pulmonary disease

Answer: b) Left ventricular failure
Explanation: Cardiogenic pulmonary edema is primarily caused by left ventricular failure, which leads to increased pressure in the pulmonary capillaries and fluid leakage into the alveoli. While fluid overload, pneumonia, and COPD can contribute to pulmonary edema, they are not the primary cause of cardiogenic pulmonary edema.

228. In the case of a tension pneumothorax, what is the initial treatment during transport?
a) Administer supplemental oxygen
b) Needle decompression
c) Initiate positive pressure ventilation
d) Administer intravenous fluids

Answer: b) Needle decompression. Explanation: The initial treatment for a tension pneumothorax during transport is needle decompression. This procedure involves inserting a large-bore needle into the pleural space to release trapped air and alleviate pressure on the mediastinum. Supplemental oxygen, positive pressure ventilation, and intravenous fluids may be used as adjunctive therapies, but needle decompression is the primary intervention for tension pneumothorax.

229. Which of the following monitoring methods is crucial for patients with respiratory emergencies during transport?
a) Continuous pulse oximetry
b) End-tidal CO2 monitoring
c) Blood pressure monitoring
d) All of the above

Answer: d) All of the above. Explanation: Continuous pulse oximetry, end-tidal CO2 monitoring, and blood pressure monitoring are all crucial for patients with respiratory emergencies during transport. These methods provide vital information on the patient's oxygenation, ventilation, and hemodynamic status, allowing for timely interventions and adjustments to treatment as needed.

230. A patient presents with chest pain, and you suspect an acute myocardial infarction (AMI). What is the most important initial diagnostic test to perform during transport?
a) Chest X-ray
b) Echocardiogram
c) 12-lead electrocardiogram (ECG)
d) CT scan of the chest

Answer: c) 12-lead electrocardiogram (ECG). Explanation: A 12-lead ECG is the most important initial diagnostic test to perform during transport for a patient presenting with chest pain and suspected AMI. The ECG can help identify ST-segment elevation myocardial infarction (STEMI) or non-ST-segment elevation myocardial infarction (NSTEMI), which are crucial for determining the appropriate treatment and management strategies.

231. Which of the following medications is part of the standard treatment for patients with chest pain due to suspected acute coronary syndrome (ACS)?
a) Nitroglycerin
b) Epinephrine
c) Albuterol
d) Furosemide

Answer: a) Nitroglycerin. Explanation: Nitroglycerin is part of the standard treatment for patients with chest pain due to suspected ACS. It acts as a vasodilator, reducing preload and afterload, which can help alleviate chest pain and improve blood flow to the myocardium. Other medications, such as epinephrine, albuterol, and furosemide, are not part of the standard treatment for suspected ACS.

232. In addition to chest pain, which of the following symptoms is commonly associated with an acute myocardial infarction (AMI)?
a) Bradycardia
b) Hypertension
c) Diaphoresis
d) Peripheral edema

Answer: c) Diaphoresis. Explanation: Diaphoresis, or excessive sweating, is a common symptom associated with an acute myocardial infarction (AMI). Other symptoms may include shortness of breath, nausea, lightheadedness, or fatigue. Bradycardia, hypertension, and peripheral edema are not typically associated with AMI.

233. What is the primary goal of prehospital management for patients with chest pain and suspected ACS?
a) Pain relief
b) Early reperfusion
c) Fluid resuscitation
d) Vasopressor administration

Answer: b) Early reperfusion. Explanation: The primary goal of prehospital management for patients with chest pain and suspected ACS is early reperfusion, which involves restoring blood flow to the ischemic myocardium. Pain relief, fluid resuscitation, and vasopressor administration may be used as adjunctive therapies, but the main objective is to minimize the extent of myocardial injury and improve patient outcomes.

234. Which of the following chest pain etiologies may present similarly to ACS but requires a different treatment approach?
a) Aortic dissection
b) Pericarditis
c) Pulmonary embolism
d) All of the above

Answer: d) All of the above. Explanation: Aortic dissection, pericarditis, and pulmonary embolism are all conditions that can present with chest pain and may mimic ACS, but each requires a different treatment approach. It is crucial for transport providers to consider alternative diagnoses and tailor treatment based on the underlying cause of the chest pain.

235. Which of the following best describes the pathophysiology of acute coronary syndromes (ACS)?
a) A sudden increase in myocardial oxygen demand
b) Plaque rupture with subsequent thrombus formation
c) Chronic inflammation of the coronary arteries
d) A vasospastic disorder affecting the coronary arteries

Answer: b) Plaque rupture with subsequent thrombus formation. Explanation: Acute coronary syndromes (ACS) are primarily caused by plaque rupture within the coronary arteries, leading to thrombus formation and subsequent myocardial ischemia. This process may result in unstable angina, non-ST elevation myocardial infarction (NSTEMI), or ST-elevation myocardial infarction (STEMI) depending on the extent of the arterial blockage and myocardial injury.

236. Which of the following ECG findings is most indicative of an ST-elevation myocardial infarction (STEMI)?
a) ST-segment depression
b) T-wave inversion
c) ST-segment elevation
d) Q-wave formation

Answer: c) ST-segment elevation. Explanation: ST-segment elevation on a 12-lead ECG is the most indicative finding of an ST-elevation myocardial infarction (STEMI). This finding suggests complete occlusion of a coronary artery and requires immediate reperfusion therapy to minimize myocardial damage and improve patient outcomes.

237. In the management of acute coronary syndromes, which of the following interventions has been shown to significantly improve patient outcomes?
a) Early reperfusion therapy
b) Administration of corticosteroids
c) Use of calcium channel blockers
d) Intravenous fluid bolus

Answer: a) Early reperfusion therapy. Explanation: Early reperfusion therapy, such as percutaneous coronary intervention (PCI) or fibrinolytic therapy, has been shown to significantly improve patient outcomes in ACS. This intervention aims to restore blood flow to the ischemic myocardium and minimize the extent of myocardial injury.

238. In the prehospital setting, which medication is often given to patients with suspected acute coronary syndromes to help reduce the risk of further thrombus formation?
a) Aspirin
b) Nitroglycerin
c) Morphine
d) Heparin

Answer: a) Aspirin. Explanation: Aspirin is an antiplatelet agent often given to patients with suspected acute coronary syndromes in the prehospital setting. It works by inhibiting platelet aggregation and reducing the risk of further thrombus formation, which can help to prevent myocardial damage and improve patient outcomes.

239. In patients with suspected STEMI, what is the recommended time from first medical contact to reperfusion therapy (e.g., percutaneous coronary intervention) to optimize patient outcomes?
a) Within 30 minutes
b) Within 60 minutes
c) Within 90 minutes
d) Within 120 minutes

Answer: c) Within 90 minutes. Explanation: In patients with suspected STEMI, the recommended time from first medical contact to reperfusion therapy (e.g., percutaneous coronary intervention) is within 90 minutes. Achieving this goal requires effective communication and coordination between prehospital providers, dispatch centers, and receiving facilities to ensure timely intervention and improve patient outcomes.

240. Which of the following is the most common cause of cardiogenic shock in patients with heart failure?
a) Acute myocardial infarction
b) Hypovolemic shock
c) Pulmonary embolism
d) Cardiac tamponade

Answer: a) Acute myocardial infarction. Explanation: Acute myocardial infarction (AMI) is the most common cause of cardiogenic shock in patients with heart failure. Cardiogenic shock occurs when the heart is unable to pump sufficient blood to meet the body's demands, leading to inadequate tissue perfusion and multi-organ dysfunction.

241. In patients experiencing heart failure exacerbation during transport, which of the following pharmacological agents is most likely to be administered to reduce preload and alleviate pulmonary congestion?
a) Beta-blockers
b) Loop diuretics
c) Angiotensin-converting enzyme (ACE) inhibitors
d) Vasopressors

Answer: b) Loop diuretics. Explanation: Loop diuretics, such as furosemide, are commonly administered to patients experiencing heart failure exacerbation during transport to reduce preload and alleviate pulmonary congestion. These medications increase urine production and help to remove excess fluid from the body, thereby reducing the workload on the heart.

242. In a patient with cardiogenic shock who is not responding to optimal medical therapy, which mechanical circulatory support device may be considered to maintain adequate tissue perfusion?
a) Intra-aortic balloon pump (IABP)
b) Extracorporeal membrane oxygenation (ECMO)
c) Ventricular assist device (VAD)
d) All of the above

Answer: d) All of the above. Explanation: In patients with cardiogenic shock who are not responding to optimal medical therapy, various mechanical circulatory support devices may be considered, including intra-aortic balloon pump (IABP), extracorporeal membrane oxygenation (ECMO), and ventricular assist devices (VADs). These devices help to maintain adequate tissue perfusion and buy time for more definitive interventions or recovery.

243. What is the primary goal of pharmacological therapy in the management of cardiogenic shock?
a) Increase afterload
b) Decrease preload
c) Improve myocardial contractility
d) Reduce heart rate

Answer: c) Improve myocardial contractility. Explanation: The primary goal of pharmacological therapy in the management of cardiogenic shock is to improve myocardial contractility. This may be achieved through the use of inotropic agents, such as dobutamine, milrinone, or dopamine, which help to enhance cardiac output and support tissue perfusion.

244. When transporting a patient with heart failure or cardiogenic shock, why is it important to collaborate with specialized cardiac care centers?
a) To ensure optimal patient outcomes
b) To obtain guidance on medication administration
c) To expedite the transfer process
d) To provide expert consultation and specialized care

Answer: d) To provide expert consultation and specialized care. Explanation: Collaboration with specialized cardiac care centers is crucial when transporting patients with heart failure or cardiogenic shock, as these facilities can provide expert consultation and specialized care, including access to advanced diagnostics, interventions, and mechanical circulatory support devices. Timely access to specialized care can significantly improve patient outcomes in these critical cases.

245. Which of the following arrhythmias is most commonly associated with hemodynamic instability and requires immediate synchronized cardioversion?
a) Ventricular tachycardia with a pulse
b) First-degree atrioventricular (AV) block
c) Atrial fibrillation
d) Sinus bradycardia

Answer: a) Ventricular tachycardia with a pulse. Explanation: Ventricular tachycardia with a pulse is a potentially life-threatening arrhythmia that is often associated with hemodynamic instability. Immediate synchronized cardioversion is required to restore normal cardiac rhythm and prevent progression to ventricular fibrillation or cardiac arrest.

246. In a patient experiencing supraventricular tachycardia (SVT) during transport, which of the following pharmacological interventions is most likely to be administered initially?
a) Adenosine
b) Amiodarone
c) Lidocaine
d) Magnesium sulfate

Answer: a) Adenosine. Explanation: Adenosine is the first-line pharmacological intervention for patients experiencing supraventricular tachycardia (SVT) during transport. Adenosine works by slowing conduction through the AV node, which can help terminate reentrant tachyarrhythmias and restore normal sinus rhythm.

247. Which type of electrical therapy is most appropriate for a patient experiencing pulseless ventricular tachycardia during transport?
a) Defibrillation
b) Synchronized cardioversion
c) Transcutaneous pacing
d) Implantable cardioverter-defibrillator (ICD) interrogation

Answer: a) Defibrillation. Explanation: Defibrillation is the most appropriate electrical therapy for a patient experiencing pulseless ventricular tachycardia during transport. Defibrillation delivers a high-energy shock to the heart, with the aim of terminating the abnormal rhythm and allowing the normal sinus rhythm to resume.

248. In a patient with atrial fibrillation and rapid ventricular response during transport, which of the following medications may be administered to control the ventricular rate?
a) Adenosine
b) Diltiazem
c) Lidocaine
d) Epinephrine

Answer: b) Diltiazem. Explanation: Diltiazem, a calcium channel blocker, may be administered to patients with atrial fibrillation and rapid ventricular response during transport to control the ventricular rate. Diltiazem slows AV node conduction, which helps to reduce the number of impulses reaching the ventricles and stabilize the patient's heart rate.

249. In which of the following situations is transcutaneous pacing most likely to be indicated during patient transport?
a) Ventricular fibrillation
b) Symptomatic sinus bradycardia unresponsive to atropine
c) Pulseless electrical activity (PEA)
d) Unstable ventricular tachycardia

Answer: b) Symptomatic sinus bradycardia unresponsive to atropine. Explanation: Transcutaneous pacing is most likely to be indicated during patient transport for symptomatic sinus bradycardia that is unresponsive to atropine. Transcutaneous pacing provides temporary pacing support by delivering electrical impulses through the chest wall to stimulate the heart, helping to maintain an adequate heart rate and perfusion until more definitive therapy can be provided.

250. A patient presents with sudden onset severe chest pain that radiates to the back. Which of the following conditions should be suspected?
a) Myocardial infarction
b) Aortic dissection
c) Pericarditis
d) Pulmonary embolism

Answer: b) Aortic dissection
Explanation: The sudden onset of severe chest pain that radiates to the back is a classic presentation of aortic dissection. Rapid diagnosis, stabilization, and transport to a specialized center for definitive care are crucial to improve patient outcomes.

251. In the context of acute aortic syndromes, which diagnostic modality is most commonly used during transport to assess for aortic dissection?
a) Chest X-ray
b) Computed tomography (CT) scan
c) Magnetic resonance imaging (MRI)
d) Bedside ultrasound

Answer: d) Bedside ultrasound
Explanation: Bedside ultrasound is the most commonly used diagnostic modality during transport to assess for aortic dissection, as it is portable and non-invasive. It can provide real-time images of the aorta, helping to identify the presence of dissection or aneurysm.

252. Which of the following medications is typically administered during transport to manage blood pressure in a patient with a suspected aortic dissection?
a) Nitroglycerin
b) Esmolol
c) Norepinephrine
d) Atropine

Answer: b) Esmolol. Explanation: Esmolol, a short-acting beta-blocker, is typically administered during transport to manage blood pressure in a patient with a suspected aortic dissection. It helps to reduce the force of ventricular contraction and heart rate, decreasing the risk of further aortic injury.

253. A patient with a suspected ruptured aortic aneurysm presents with hypotension and a pulsatile abdominal mass. Which of the following interventions should be prioritized during transport?
a) Aggressive fluid resuscitation
b) Permissive hypotension
c) Administration of vasopressors
d) Immediate surgical intervention

Answer: b) Permissive hypotension

Explanation: Permissive hypotension should be prioritized during transport for a patient with a suspected ruptured aortic aneurysm. Aggressive fluid resuscitation can increase blood pressure and worsen the bleeding, while vasopressors may have a similar effect. Permissive hypotension involves maintaining a lower-than-normal blood pressure to minimize the risk of further hemorrhage while ensuring adequate organ perfusion.

254. What is the definitive treatment for a patient with an acute aortic syndrome, such as aortic dissection or ruptured aortic aneurysm?
a) Pharmacological management
b) Percutaneous coronary intervention (PCI)
c) Surgical repair or endovascular intervention
d) Implantation of a ventricular assist device (VAD)

Answer: c) Surgical repair or endovascular intervention

Explanation: The definitive treatment for a patient with an acute aortic syndrome, such as aortic dissection or ruptured aortic aneurysm, is surgical repair or endovascular intervention. Rapid diagnosis, stabilization, and transport to a specialized center for definitive care are essential to improve patient outcomes.

255. A patient presents with sudden dyspnea, wheezing, and coughing. The patient has a known history of asthma. Which of the following medications should be administered first?
a) Inhaled short-acting beta-agonist (SABA)
b) Intravenous corticosteroids
c) Inhaled anticholinergics
d) Intravenous magnesium sulfate

Answer: a) Inhaled short-acting beta-agonist (SABA)

Explanation: In a patient with sudden dyspnea, wheezing, and coughing, and a known history of asthma, the first-line treatment is an inhaled short-acting beta-agonist (SABA), such as albuterol. SABAs provide rapid bronchodilation, helping to relieve symptoms and improve airflow.

256. A patient with a history of chronic obstructive pulmonary disease (COPD) presents with increased dyspnea, sputum production, and purulent sputum. Which intervention is most appropriate for managing a COPD exacerbation?
a) Administer high-flow oxygen therapy
b) Initiate noninvasive positive pressure ventilation (NIPPV)
c) Administer nebulized ipratropium bromide
d) Perform endotracheal intubation

Answer: b) Initiate noninvasive positive pressure ventilation (NIPPV)

Explanation: For a patient with a COPD exacerbation, initiating noninvasive positive pressure ventilation (NIPPV) is the most appropriate intervention. NIPPV helps to improve oxygenation, reduce the work of breathing, and decrease the need for intubation.

257. A patient in respiratory distress presents with pink, frothy sputum and crackles on lung auscultation. Which of the following conditions is most likely, and what is the first-line treatment?
a) Pulmonary edema; administer nitroglycerin
b) Pneumothorax; perform needle decompression
c) Asthma exacerbation; administer inhaled short-acting beta-agonist
d) COPD exacerbation; administer inhaled anticholinergics

Answer: a) Pulmonary edema; administer nitroglycerin
Explanation: The presence of pink, frothy sputum and crackles on lung auscultation suggest pulmonary edema. The first-line treatment for pulmonary edema is the administration of nitroglycerin, which helps to reduce preload, afterload, and pulmonary congestion.

258. A patient presents with sudden onset dyspnea and decreased breath sounds on one side of the chest. Which condition should be suspected, and what is the initial treatment?
a) Pneumothorax; perform needle decompression
b) Pulmonary embolism; administer anticoagulants
c) Acute respiratory distress syndrome (ARDS); initiate lung-protective ventilation
d) Asthma exacerbation; administer inhaled short-acting beta-agonist

Answer: a) Pneumothorax; perform needle decompression
Explanation: The sudden onset of dyspnea and decreased breath sounds on one side of the chest suggest pneumothorax. The initial treatment for a tension pneumothorax is needle decompression to relieve the pressure and allow for lung re-expansion.

259. Which of the following respiratory emergencies is primarily managed with anticoagulant therapy?
a) Acute respiratory distress syndrome (ARDS)
b) Pulmonary embolism
c) Pneumothorax
d) Pulmonary edema

Answer: b) Pulmonary embolism
Explanation: Pulmonary embolism is primarily managed with anticoagulant therapy, which helps to prevent clot formation and propagation.

260. Which of the following clinical presentations is most consistent with an ST-elevation myocardial infarction (STEMI)?
a) Isolated shortness of breath
b) Chest pain relieved by antacids
c) Chest pain radiating to the left arm, associated with diaphoresis and nausea
d) Sharp, pleuritic chest pain worsened by deep breaths

Answer: c) Chest pain radiating to the left arm, associated with diaphoresis and nausea
Explanation: Chest pain radiating to the left arm, associated with diaphoresis and nausea, is a classic presentation of a STEMI. The pain in STEMI is usually severe, crushing, or pressure-like and is not relieved by antacids or positional changes.

261. In the prehospital setting, what is the most important diagnostic tool for identifying an acute coronary syndrome?
a) Blood tests for cardiac biomarkers
b) Chest X-ray
c) 12-lead electrocardiogram (ECG)
d) Echocardiography

Answer: c) 12-lead electrocardiogram (ECG)
Explanation: A 12-lead ECG is the most important diagnostic tool for identifying acute coronary syndromes in the prehospital setting. It allows for the rapid detection of ST-segment changes, which can help differentiate between STEMI and NSTEMI, guiding appropriate treatment and destination decisions.

262. What is the first-line pharmacological treatment for patients presenting with chest pain suggestive of an acute coronary syndrome?
a) Nitroglycerin
b) Beta-blockers
c) Morphine
d) Aspirin

Answer: d) Aspirin
Explanation: Aspirin is the first-line pharmacological treatment for patients presenting with chest pain suggestive of an acute coronary syndrome. It has antiplatelet effects, reducing clot formation and propagation, and has been shown to improve outcomes in patients with ACS.

263. Which of the following interventions is contraindicated in a patient with a suspected STEMI?
a) Oxygen therapy
b) Administration of beta-blockers
c) Intravenous fibrinolytic therapy
d) Immediate percutaneous coronary intervention (PCI)

Answer: c) Intravenous fibrinolytic therapy
Explanation: Intravenous fibrinolytic therapy is contraindicated in patients with a suspected STEMI. The preferred reperfusion strategy for STEMI patients is primary percutaneous coronary intervention (PCI) performed at a specialized cardiac care center, as it has been shown to be more effective than fibrinolytic therapy in reducing mortality and morbidity.

264. What is the recommended time frame for door-to-balloon time in patients presenting with STEMI?
a) Less than 60 minutes
b) Less than 90 minutes
c) Less than 120 minutes
d) Less than 180 minutes

Answer: b) Less than 90 minutes. Explanation: The recommended time frame for door-to-balloon time in patients presenting with STEMI is less than 90 minutes. This means that from the time the patient arrives at the hospital to the time the blocked coronary artery is opened via percutaneous coronary intervention (PCI), no more than 90 minutes should elapse. This goal emphasizes the importance of early recognition, ECG monitoring, and coordination with specialized cardiac care centers.

265. What is the most crucial factor in determining the prognosis and long-term outcomes of a patient with acute ischemic stroke?
a) The severity of the initial neurological deficit
b) The patient's age
c) The time from symptom onset to treatment initiation
d) The presence of comorbidities

Answer: c) The time from symptom onset to treatment initiation
Explanation: The time from symptom onset to treatment initiation is the most crucial factor in determining the prognosis and long-term outcomes of a patient with acute ischemic stroke. Rapid assessment, timely transportation, and appropriate management can significantly improve outcomes by minimizing the extent of brain injury.

266. Which of the following assessment tools is recommended for prehospital healthcare providers to screen for a possible stroke?
a) Glasgow Coma Scale (GCS)
b) Cincinnati Prehospital Stroke Scale (CPSS)
c) Modified Rankin Scale (mRS)
d) National Institutes of Health Stroke Scale (NIHSS)

Answer: b) Cincinnati Prehospital Stroke Scale (CPSS)
Explanation: The Cincinnati Prehospital Stroke Scale (CPSS) is a quick and straightforward assessment tool designed for prehospital healthcare providers to screen for a possible stroke. The CPSS evaluates facial droop, arm drift, and speech abnormalities, which are classic symptoms of stroke.

267. Which of the following is the most common type of stroke?
a) Hemorrhagic stroke
b) Ischemic stroke
c) Subarachnoid hemorrhage
d) Transient ischemic attack (TIA)

Answer: b) Ischemic stroke. Explanation: Ischemic stroke is the most common type of stroke, accounting for approximately 87% of all stroke cases. It occurs when a blood clot blocks blood flow to a part of the brain, depriving brain cells of oxygen and nutrients.

268. What is the primary pharmacological treatment for patients with acute ischemic stroke who meet specific criteria?
a) Antiplatelet agents
b) Anticoagulants
c) Intravenous tissue plasminogen activator (tPA)
d) Calcium channel blockers

Answer: c) Intravenous tissue plasminogen activator (tPA). Explanation: Intravenous tissue plasminogen activator (tPA) is the primary pharmacological treatment for patients with acute ischemic stroke who meet specific criteria. It works by dissolving the blood clot responsible for the stroke, restoring blood flow to the affected area of the brain.

269. What is the most appropriate course of action for a healthcare provider when managing a patient experiencing a generalized tonic-clonic seizure?
a) Administer intravenous benzodiazepines immediately
b) Restrain the patient to prevent injury
c) Insert an oral airway to maintain airway patency
d) Protect the patient's head and ensure a safe environment

Answer: d) Protect the patient's head and ensure a safe environment
Explanation: The most appropriate course of action for a healthcare provider when managing a patient experiencing a generalized tonic-clonic seizure is to protect the patient's head and ensure a safe environment. This prevents injury during the seizure. Restraining the patient and inserting an oral airway are not recommended, as they may cause harm. Benzodiazepines may be considered if the seizure lasts longer than 5 minutes or the patient has multiple seizures without regaining consciousness.

270. Which of the following is the most common precipitating factor for diabetic ketoacidosis (DKA)?
a) Inadequate insulin administration
b) Alcohol consumption
c) Overeating carbohydrates
d) Overexertion during exercise

Answer: a) Inadequate insulin administration
Explanation: Inadequate insulin administration is the most common precipitating factor for diabetic ketoacidosis (DKA). When insulin levels are insufficient, the body cannot effectively use glucose for energy and starts breaking down fats, leading to the production of ketones and subsequent acidosis.

271. Which clinical feature differentiates hyperglycemic hyperosmolar state (HHS) from diabetic ketoacidosis (DKA)?
a) Hyperglycemia
b) Dehydration
c) Acidosis
d) Ketonuria

Answer: c) Acidosis
Explanation: Acidosis differentiates hyperglycemic hyperosmolar state (HHS) from diabetic ketoacidosis (DKA). While both conditions present with hyperglycemia and dehydration, DKA is characterized by acidosis and ketonuria, whereas HHS typically has minimal or no ketonuria and a near-normal blood pH.

272. A patient with type 1 diabetes presents with a blood glucose level of 55 mg/dL. What is the most appropriate initial treatment?
a) Administer intravenous insulin
b) Give oral glucose gel or a sugary drink
c) Administer intravenous dextrose
d) Provide subcutaneous glucagon

Answer: b) Give oral glucose gel or a sugary drink. Explanation: For a conscious patient with a blood glucose level of 55 mg/dL, the most appropriate initial treatment is to give oral glucose gel or a sugary drink. This will help rapidly raise blood glucose levels. Other interventions such as intravenous insulin, intravenous dextrose, and subcutaneous glucagon are not indicated in this scenario.

273. Which laboratory finding is most indicative of diabetic ketoacidosis (DKA)?
a) Blood glucose > 250 mg/dL
b) Serum bicarbonate < 18 mEq/L
c) Positive serum ketones
d) All of the above

Answer: d) All of the above. Explanation: All of the listed laboratory findings (blood glucose > 250 mg/dL, serum bicarbonate < 18 mEq/L, and positive serum ketones) are indicative of diabetic ketoacidosis (DKA). These lab values help differentiate DKA from other conditions such as hyperglycemic hyperosmolar state (HHS) and simple hyperglycemia.

274. Which of the following is a primary treatment goal for patients with hyperglycemic hyperosmolar state (HHS)?
a) Aggressive insulin therapy
b) Rapid rehydration with isotonic fluids
c) Immediate correction of electrolyte imbalances
d) Quick administration of potassium supplements

Answer: b) Rapid rehydration with isotonic fluids. Explanation: Rapid rehydration with isotonic fluids is a primary treatment goal for patients with hyperglycemic hyperosmolar state (HHS). Rehydration helps correct severe dehydration, improve renal function, and lower blood glucose levels. Insulin therapy, electrolyte correction, and potassium supplementation are also important aspects of HHS management, but they are secondary to rehydration.

275. Which of the following is the most appropriate first-line treatment for a patient with suspected opioid overdose?
a) Administer activated charcoal
b) Provide high-flow oxygen
c) Administer naloxone
d) Perform gastric lavage

Answer: c) Administer naloxone. Explanation: Naloxone is the most appropriate first-line treatment for a patient with suspected opioid overdose. It is an opioid antagonist that rapidly reverses the respiratory depression and other effects of opioid overdose. Activated charcoal, high-flow oxygen, and gastric lavage may be considered in certain cases, but they are not the primary treatments for opioid overdose.

276. A patient presents with altered mental status, seizures, and metabolic acidosis after ingesting an unknown substance. What is the most likely cause of the patient's symptoms?
a) Organophosphate poisoning
b) Carbon monoxide poisoning
c) Methanol or ethylene glycol poisoning
d) Cyanide poisoning

Answer: c) Methanol or ethylene glycol poisoning
Explanation: Methanol or ethylene glycol poisoning is the most likely cause of the patient's symptoms, as ingestion of these substances can lead to altered mental status, seizures, and metabolic acidosis. Organophosphate poisoning, carbon monoxide poisoning, and cyanide poisoning can also cause altered mental status, but they have different clinical presentations and are less likely to cause the combination of symptoms described.

277. In the case of a snakebite from a venomous snake, which intervention should be avoided?
a) Immobilizing the affected limb
b) Applying a tourniquet
c) Administering antivenom, if indicated
d) Transporting the patient to a medical facility

Answer: b) Applying a tourniquet
Explanation: Applying a tourniquet should be avoided in the case of a venomous snakebite, as it can cause localized tissue damage and worsen the effects of the venom. Immobilizing the affected limb, administering antivenom (if indicated), and transporting the patient to a medical facility are appropriate interventions.

278. Which treatment is indicated for a patient with severe carbon monoxide poisoning?
a) Administering 100% oxygen via a non-rebreather mask
b) Giving intravenous fluids
c) Administering activated charcoal
d) Providing benzodiazepines for seizures

Answer: a) Administering 100% oxygen via a non-rebreather mask
Explanation: Administering 100% oxygen via a non-rebreather mask is the primary treatment for severe carbon monoxide poisoning. This intervention helps to displace carbon monoxide from hemoglobin, allowing the patient's tissues to receive oxygen. Intravenous fluids, activated charcoal, and benzodiazepines may be indicated for other toxicological emergencies, but they are not the primary treatments for carbon monoxide poisoning.

279. Which of the following is a key principle in managing most toxic exposures?
a) Providing supportive care
b) Administering a specific antidote
c) Inducing vomiting
d) Performing gastric lavage

Answer: a) Providing supportive care
Explanation: Providing supportive care is a key principle in managing most toxic exposures. Supportive care focuses on stabilizing the patient, maintaining airway patency, and ensuring adequate oxygenation and circulation. While specific antidotes may be used for certain exposures, they are not applicable in all cases. Inducing vomiting and performing gastric lavage are outdated practices and are not recommended in most cases.

280. What is the key difference between heat exhaustion and heatstroke?
a) The presence of muscle cramps
b) Core body temperature
c) The level of dehydration
d) The presence of altered mental status

Answer: d) The presence of altered mental status
Explanation: The key difference between heat exhaustion and heatstroke is the presence of altered mental status. Heat exhaustion is characterized by symptoms such as weakness, dizziness, and excessive sweating but with normal mental status. Heatstroke, on the other hand, presents with altered mental status, indicating a more severe and life-threatening condition.

281. A patient with severe hypothermia presents with a slow and weak pulse. Which of the following should be avoided during the management of this patient?
a) Passive rewarming
b) Administering warm intravenous fluids
c) Applying direct heat to the extremities
d) Monitoring core body temperature

Answer: c) Applying direct heat to the extremities. Explanation: Applying direct heat to the extremities should be avoided in patients with severe hypothermia, as it may cause peripheral vasodilation, leading to a decrease in the core body temperature. Passive rewarming, administering warm intravenous fluids, and monitoring core body temperature are all appropriate interventions for severe hypothermia.

282. Which of the following is an early sign of frostbite?
a) White, waxy skin
b) Red and swollen skin
c) Blue-gray skin
d) Blackened skin and tissue loss

Answer: b) Red and swollen skin. Explanation: Red and swollen skin is an early sign of frostbite, indicating the beginning stages of cold injury. As frostbite progresses, the skin may become white and waxy, then blue-gray, and eventually blackened with tissue loss in severe cases.

283. In a patient with suspected heatstroke, which intervention is crucial for preventing further complications?
a) Administering intravenous fluids
b) Rapidly cooling the patient
c) Providing supplemental oxygen
d) Administering antipyretics

Answer: b) Rapidly cooling the patient. Explanation: Rapidly cooling the patient is crucial for preventing further complications in a patient with suspected heatstroke. This can be achieved through methods such as cold water immersion or evaporative cooling. While administering intravenous fluids and providing supplemental oxygen may also be beneficial, cooling the patient takes priority. Antipyretics are not effective in treating heatstroke, as the underlying cause is not fever but rather an inability to regulate body temperature.

284. Which of the following is an appropriate management strategy for a patient with mild hypothermia?
a) Immersing the patient in warm water
b) Applying heated blankets to the torso
c) Administering warmed intravenous fluids
d) Initiating active external rewarming

Answer: b) Applying heated blankets to the torso
Explanation: Applying heated blankets to the patient's torso is an appropriate management strategy for mild hypothermia. This approach provides gentle, controlled warming of the patient's core. Immersion in warm water and administering warmed intravenous fluids are more aggressive rewarming techniques reserved for moderate to severe hypothermia, while active external rewarming may be too aggressive for mild cases.

285. What is the primary cause of death in drowning incidents?
a) Hypothermia
b) Hypoxia
c) Cardiac arrhythmia
d) Fluid aspiration

Answer: b) Hypoxia. Explanation: Hypoxia is the primary cause of death in drowning incidents. Oxygen deprivation due to water entering the lungs and disrupting gas exchange leads to hypoxia, which can cause multi-organ failure and ultimately death if not promptly addressed.

286. In a near-drowning incident, which of the following complications is most likely to develop in the first 24 hours?
a) Hypothermia
b) Pulmonary edema
c) Seizures
d) Electrolyte imbalances

Answer: b) Pulmonary edema. Explanation: Pulmonary edema is the most likely complication to develop within the first 24 hours following a near-drowning incident. It results from fluid accumulation in the lungs due to the damage caused by the drowning process, which can impair gas exchange and cause respiratory distress.

287. Which of the following is the most appropriate initial intervention for a patient who has been rescued from a drowning incident and is unresponsive but has a pulse?
a) Provide supplemental oxygen
b) Begin chest compressions
c) Initiate active rewarming
d) Perform a jaw-thrust maneuver

Answer: a) Provide supplemental oxygen. Explanation: Providing supplemental oxygen is the most appropriate initial intervention for an unresponsive patient with a pulse following a drowning incident. Oxygen should be administered to reverse hypoxia, which is the primary cause of morbidity and mortality in drowning cases. Other interventions, such as chest compressions or rewarming, may be necessary depending on the patient's condition but are not the initial priority.

288. In a drowning incident, which of the following factors has the greatest impact on long-term neurological outcomes?
a) Water temperature
b) Duration of submersion
c) Age of the patient
d) Presence of a pulse upon rescue

Answer: b) Duration of submersion
Explanation: The duration of submersion has the greatest impact on long-term neurological outcomes in drowning incidents. Prolonged submersion increases the severity of hypoxia and the likelihood of irreversible brain damage. While factors such as water temperature, patient age, and the presence of a pulse upon rescue may also influence outcomes, submersion duration is the most critical determinant.

289. Which of the following is NOT a recommended intervention for managing a drowning patient with hypothermia?
a) Passive external rewarming
b) Active internal rewarming with warmed intravenous fluids
c) Administration of vasopressors
d) Active external rewarming with a heating blanket

Answer: c) Administration of vasopressors
Explanation: Administration of vasopressors is not a recommended intervention for managing a drowning patient with hypothermia. Vasopressors can cause peripheral vasoconstriction, which may exacerbate hypothermia by reducing blood flow to the extremities. Instead, interventions such as passive external rewarming, active internal rewarming with warmed intravenous fluids, or active external rewarming with a heating blanket can be used to manage hypothermia in drowning patients.

290. Which of the following venomous snakebites is associated with the development of neurotoxic symptoms, such as ptosis, difficulty swallowing, and muscle weakness?
a) Rattlesnake
b) Copperhead
c) Coral snake
d) Water moccasin

Answer: c) Coral snake
Explanation: Coral snake bites are associated with the development of neurotoxic symptoms. The venom of coral snakes contains potent neurotoxins that can cause muscle paralysis, respiratory failure, and other neurological symptoms. Other snakebites, such as those from rattlesnakes, copperheads, and water moccasins, are more likely to cause local tissue damage and coagulopathy.

291. A patient who has been bitten by an insect presents with an expanding target-shaped rash. Which insect is most likely responsible for the bite?
a) Tick
b) Mosquito
c) Spider
d) Bee

Answer: a) Tick
Explanation: The expanding target-shaped rash, also known as erythema migrans, is characteristic of a tick bite and is a hallmark of Lyme disease. Ticks can transmit the bacterium Borrelia burgdorferi, which causes Lyme disease. The rash typically appears within a week after the bite and expands outward from the bite site.

292. What is the appropriate initial treatment for a patient stung by a jellyfish?
a) Washing the affected area with freshwater
b) Rinsing the area with vinegar
c) Applying ice to the affected area
d) Rubbing the area with sand

Answer: b) Rinsing the area with vinegar
Explanation: Rinsing the area with vinegar is the appropriate initial treatment for a patient stung by a jellyfish. Vinegar can help to neutralize the nematocysts (stinging cells) and prevent further venom release. Washing the affected area with freshwater or rubbing it with sand can cause additional nematocysts to release venom, worsening the sting.

293. Which of the following is a common systemic reaction to a bee sting?
a) Anaphylaxis
b) Acute renal failure
c) Hemolytic anemia
d) Coagulopathy

Answer: a) Anaphylaxis
Explanation: Anaphylaxis is a common systemic reaction to a bee sting, particularly in individuals with a known allergy to bee venom. Anaphylaxis can cause symptoms such as difficulty breathing, swelling of the face or throat, and a rapid drop in blood pressure. It requires immediate medical intervention, including the administration of epinephrine.

294. nIn the event of a venomous snakebite, which of the following interventions should be avoided?
a) Immobilizing the affected limb
b) Applying a tourniquet above the bite site
c) Administering antivenom
d) Keeping the patient calm and still

Answer: b) Applying a tourniquet above the bite site
Explanation: Applying a tourniquet above the bite site should be avoided in the event of a venomous snakebite. Tourniquets can restrict blood flow and cause additional tissue damage. Instead, the affected limb should be immobilized, and the patient should be kept calm and still while awaiting medical care. Antivenom may be administered as appropriate to neutralize the venom and reduce complications.

295. What is the most effective initial strategy for preventing acute mountain sickness (AMS)?
a) Taking acetazolamide before ascent
b) Ascending rapidly to acclimatize more quickly
c) Gradual ascent with proper acclimatization
d) Drinking large amounts of water

Answer: c) Gradual ascent with proper acclimatization
Explanation: The most effective initial strategy for preventing acute mountain sickness (AMS) is a gradual ascent with proper acclimatization. This allows the body to adapt to the lower oxygen levels at high altitudes. Rapid ascent and inadequate acclimatization can increase the risk of developing AMS.

296. A patient presents with severe headache, nausea, and ataxia at high altitude. Which altitude-related illness is most likely?
a) Acute mountain sickness (AMS)
b) High-altitude cerebral edema (HACE)
c) High-altitude pulmonary edema (HAPE)
d) Chronic mountain sickness (CMS)

Answer: b) High-altitude cerebral edema (HACE)
Explanation: High-altitude cerebral edema (HACE) is most likely the cause of the patient's symptoms. HACE is a severe form of acute mountain sickness and is characterized by severe headache, nausea, vomiting, ataxia, and altered mental status. It is a life-threatening condition that requires immediate descent and medical intervention.

297. Which medication is commonly used as a prophylactic measure to prevent acute mountain sickness (AMS) in high-risk individuals?
a) Acetazolamide
b) Ibuprofen
c) Nifedipine
d) Furosemide

Answer: a) Acetazolamide
Explanation: Acetazolamide is commonly used as a prophylactic measure to prevent acute mountain sickness (AMS) in high-risk individuals. It works by stimulating ventilation and increasing the amount of oxygen in the bloodstream, helping the body to acclimatize more effectively at high altitudes.

298. What is the primary treatment for high-altitude pulmonary edema (HAPE)?
a) Supplemental oxygen
b) Immediate descent to a lower altitude
c) Administration of nifedipine
d) Intravenous fluids

Answer: b) Immediate descent to a lower altitude. Explanation: The primary treatment for high-altitude pulmonary edema (HAPE) is immediate descent to a lower altitude. Descent helps alleviate the hypoxic conditions that contribute to the development of HAPE. Supplemental oxygen, nifedipine, and other supportive measures can be used to manage symptoms and stabilize the patient during the descent.

299. A group of climbers is ascending a high-altitude mountain, and one of them begins to exhibit signs of acute mountain sickness (AMS). What is the most appropriate initial action to take?
a) Administer acetazolamide immediately
b) Continue ascending but at a slower pace
c) Descend to a lower altitude
d) Rest at the current altitude for 24 hours

Answer: d) Rest at the current altitude for 24 hours
Explanation: If a climber begins to exhibit signs of acute mountain sickness (AMS), the most appropriate initial action is to rest at the current altitude for 24 hours. This allows the body to acclimatize further and may alleviate the symptoms of AMS. If symptoms worsen or do not improve after 24 hours, descending to a lower altitude is recommended.

300. In the primary survey of a trauma patient, what is the primary focus during the "C" component (Circulation)?
a) Evaluating the quality of peripheral pulses
b) Assessing for internal and external bleeding
c) Obtaining a blood pressure measurement
d) Initiating intravenous fluid resuscitation

Answer: b) Assessing for internal and external bleeding
Explanation: During the "C" component (Circulation) of the primary survey, the primary focus is on assessing for internal and external bleeding. Rapid identification and control of life-threatening bleeding is crucial to increase the patient's chance of survival.

301. Which of the following signs is the most concerning in a patient with a suspected traumatic brain injury (TBI)?
a) Mild headache
b) Retrograde amnesia
c) Unequal pupil size
d) Mild dizziness

Answer: c) Unequal pupil size
Explanation: Unequal pupil size (anisocoria) is the most concerning sign in a patient with a suspected traumatic brain injury (TBI), as it may indicate increased intracranial pressure, brainstem injury, or other serious neurological issues. Immediate medical attention and intervention are necessary.

302. A patient with blunt chest trauma presents with absent breath sounds on the left side, tracheal deviation to the right, and jugular vein distension. What is the most likely diagnosis?
a) Hemothorax
b) Tension pneumothorax
c) Flail chest
d) Cardiac tamponade

Answer: b) Tension pneumothorax
Explanation: The patient's presentation of absent breath sounds on the left side, tracheal deviation to the right, and jugular vein distension are suggestive of a tension pneumothorax. This life-threatening condition requires immediate intervention, such as needle decompression, to relieve the pressure in the pleural space.

303. Which of the following interventions is most critical for a patient with a suspected spinal cord injury?
a) Administration of high-flow oxygen
b) Spinal immobilization
c) Intravenous fluid resuscitation
d) Pain management

Answer: b) Spinal immobilization
Explanation: Spinal immobilization is the most critical intervention for a patient with a suspected spinal cord injury. It helps to prevent further injury and potential neurological damage during assessment, stabilization, and transportation.

304. When assessing a patient with a suspected musculoskeletal injury, which of the following steps should be prioritized?
a) Assessing distal pulse, motor function, and sensation
b) Splinting the injured extremity
c) Administering pain medication
d) Applying ice to the injury site

Answer: a) Assessing distal pulse, motor function, and sensation
Explanation: Assessing distal pulse, motor function, and sensation should be prioritized when evaluating a patient with a suspected musculoskeletal injury. This assessment helps to determine the severity of the injury and the need for additional interventions or transportation to an appropriate healthcare facility for definitive care.

305. Which of the following factors should be considered when assessing a pediatric patient's airway?
a) Children have relatively larger heads and tongues compared to adults.
b) Children have shorter necks, making intubation easier.
c) Children have well-developed neck muscles, providing extra support.
d) Children's airways are more rigid than those of adults.

Answer: a) Children have relatively larger heads and tongues compared to adults.
Explanation: When assessing a pediatric patient's airway, it is important to consider that children have relatively larger heads and tongues compared to adults. This anatomical difference may impact airway management techniques and increase the risk of airway obstruction.

306. What is a key principle when assessing pain in geriatric patients?
a) Geriatric patients are less likely to report pain.
b) Geriatric patients typically experience less pain due to decreased nerve function.
c) Geriatric patients always require higher doses of pain medication.
d) Geriatric patients are more likely to exaggerate their pain levels.

Answer: a) Geriatric patients are less likely to report pain.
Explanation: Geriatric patients may be less likely to report pain due to various factors, such as stoicism, cognitive impairment, or fear of being a burden. Healthcare providers should use a comprehensive approach to assess pain in geriatric patients, considering both verbal and nonverbal cues.

307. In pediatric patients, which of the following signs may indicate compensated shock?
a) Bradycardia
b) Mottled skin
c) Delayed capillary refill
d) Hypotension

Answer: c) Delayed capillary refill

Explanation: Delayed capillary refill is a sign of compensated shock in pediatric patients. Children may initially compensate for shock by increasing their heart rate and maintaining blood pressure, but as shock progresses, perfusion decreases, leading to delayed capillary refill.

308. When assessing a geriatric patient's mental status, which of the following factors should be considered?
a) Baseline cognitive function
b) Time of day
c) Presence of sensory impairments
d) All of the above

Answer: d) All of the above

Explanation: When assessing a geriatric patient's mental status, it is important to consider their baseline cognitive function, time of day (as confusion may be more prominent at night), and the presence of sensory impairments (such as hearing or vision loss) that may impact their ability to communicate and understand.

309. In which of the following scenarios would the use of the Pediatric Assessment Triangle (PAT) be most appropriate?
a) Evaluating a pediatric patient with a suspected fracture
b) Assessing a pediatric patient with difficulty breathing
c) Calculating the correct medication dosage for a pediatric patient
d) Performing a neurological examination on a pediatric patient

Answer: b) Assessing a pediatric patient with difficulty breathing

Explanation: The Pediatric Assessment Triangle (PAT) is a rapid assessment tool used to evaluate a child's appearance, work of breathing, and circulation to the skin. It is most appropriate for assessing pediatric patients with difficulty breathing, as it helps to quickly identify signs of respiratory distress and guide interventions.

310. A pregnant patient at 34 weeks gestation presents with sudden onset of severe, constant abdominal pain and vaginal bleeding. What is the most likely diagnosis?
a) Placenta previa
b) Abruptio placentae
c) Uterine rupture
d) Preterm labor

Answer: b) Abruptio placentae

Explanation: Abruptio placentae is the premature separation of the placenta from the uterus, and it often presents with sudden onset of severe, constant abdominal pain and vaginal bleeding. This condition is a medical emergency and requires prompt intervention.

311. When assisting with an emergency childbirth, which of the following interventions is appropriate during the delivery of the baby's head?
a) Apply gentle upward pressure on the baby's head.
b) Apply gentle downward pressure on the baby's head.
c) Apply fundal pressure to assist with delivery.
d) Encourage the mother to push forcefully.

Answer: a) Apply gentle upward pressure on the baby's head.
Explanation: During the delivery of the baby's head, applying gentle upward pressure can help to guide the head out and prevent rapid expulsion, reducing the risk of perineal tearing.

312. A postpartum patient is experiencing a significant amount of vaginal bleeding. What is the first step in managing this situation?
a) Administer IV fluids.
b) Perform a bimanual uterine massage.
c) Encourage the patient to breastfeed.
d) Administer oxytocin.

Answer: b) Perform a bimanual uterine massage.
Explanation: The first step in managing significant postpartum bleeding is to perform a bimanual uterine massage, which can help stimulate uterine contractions and reduce bleeding. Further interventions may be necessary depending on the patient's response.

313. Which of the following is a potential complication of eclampsia?
a) Hyperglycemia
b) Pulmonary edema
c) Bradycardia
d) Hypothermia

Answer: b) Pulmonary edema
Explanation: Eclampsia is a severe complication of preeclampsia and is characterized by seizures. Pulmonary edema is a potential complication of eclampsia due to fluid shifts, increased vascular permeability, and decreased oncotic pressure.

314. A patient presents with lower abdominal pain, vaginal bleeding, and a positive pregnancy test. The patient is hemodynamically stable. What is the most likely diagnosis?
a) Ectopic pregnancy
b) Spontaneous abortion
c) Placenta previa
d) Abruptio placentae

Answer: a) Ectopic pregnancy
Explanation: Ectopic pregnancy occurs when the fertilized egg implants outside the uterus, typically in the fallopian tube. It presents with lower abdominal pain, vaginal bleeding, and a positive pregnancy test. While the patient may initially be hemodynamically stable, an ectopic pregnancy can lead to life-threatening bleeding if not diagnosed and treated promptly.

315. Which of the following communication techniques is most appropriate when dealing with a patient experiencing a mental health crisis?
a) Speak loudly and firmly to establish authority.
b) Use closed-ended questions to gather information quickly.
c) Maintain direct eye contact to show attentiveness.
d) Use active listening and empathetic responses to foster rapport.

Answer: d) Use active listening and empathetic responses to foster rapport.
Explanation: When dealing with a patient experiencing a mental health crisis, it is important to use active listening and empathetic responses to establish rapport and build trust. This can help the patient feel heard and understood, making them more likely to cooperate with care.

316. What is the primary goal of de-escalation techniques when managing a patient in a mental health crisis?
a) To take control of the situation
b) To ensure the safety of the patient, healthcare providers, and others
c) To establish a diagnosis as quickly as possible
d) To convince the patient to agree with the healthcare provider

Answer: b) To ensure the safety of the patient, healthcare providers, and others
Explanation: The primary goal of de-escalation techniques is to ensure the safety of the patient, healthcare providers, and others involved in the situation. This can be achieved by calming the patient, reducing agitation, and preventing aggressive behavior.

317. When assessing a patient with a potential mental health crisis, which of the following should be a priority?
a) Evaluating the patient's mental status and level of agitation
b) Obtaining a detailed medical and psychiatric history
c) Assessing for signs of substance use or withdrawal
d) Identifying potential safety risks and triggers

Answer: d) Identifying potential safety risks and triggers
Explanation: While all of these factors are important in assessing a patient with a mental health crisis, identifying potential safety risks and triggers should be a priority. This can help inform appropriate interventions, manage the situation effectively, and prevent harm to the patient or others.

318. Which of the following is an appropriate intervention for a patient experiencing a panic attack?
a) Administering a sedative medication
b) Encouraging the patient to take slow, deep breaths
c) Providing reassurance that their symptoms are not life-threatening
d) Both b and c

Answer: d) Both b and c
Explanation: For a patient experiencing a panic attack, interventions should focus on calming the patient and providing reassurance. Encouraging slow, deep breaths can help regulate the patient's breathing, while providing reassurance that their symptoms are not life-threatening can help alleviate anxiety.

319. A patient experiencing a mental health crisis is refusing to cooperate with healthcare providers. What is the most appropriate initial response?
a) Insist on cooperation and explain the consequences of noncompliance.
b) Attempt to establish rapport by discussing the patient's interests or concerns.
c) Immediately restrain the patient for their safety and the safety of others.
d) Administer a sedative medication to calm the patient.

Answer: b) Attempt to establish rapport by discussing the patient's interests or concerns.
Explanation: The most appropriate initial response to a patient refusing to cooperate is to attempt to establish rapport by discussing the patient's interests or concerns. This can help build trust and make the patient more willing to cooperate with care. Restraining or sedating the patient should be considered only if other approaches fail and there is an imminent risk to the patient or others.

320. When providing emergency care to a patient with a hearing impairment, which communication strategy is most effective?
a) Speak loudly and slowly, while maintaining eye contact.
b) Utilize written communication or a communication device if available.
c) Use gestures and body language to convey important information.
d) Rely on a family member to relay all information.

Answer: b) Utilize written communication or a communication device if available.
Explanation: When communicating with a patient with a hearing impairment, written communication or a communication device can be the most effective method. This ensures clear communication and allows the patient to fully understand the information being conveyed.

321. When assessing a patient with a cognitive disability, which of the following strategies should be employed?
a) Avoid using medical jargon or complex language.
b) Speak to the patient as if they were a child.
c) Focus on the caregiver's perspective rather than the patient's.
d) Assume the patient cannot understand the situation or instructions.

Answer: a) Avoid using medical jargon or complex language.
Explanation: When assessing a patient with a cognitive disability, it is important to avoid using medical jargon or complex language. Instead, use clear and simple language that the patient can understand. Avoid speaking to the patient as if they were a child, and always address the patient directly rather than focusing on the caregiver's perspective.

322. A patient with a sensory disability, such as blindness or low vision, may require which of the following modifications in care?
a) Greater reliance on verbal communication to convey information
b) Immediate sedation to prevent anxiety or agitation
c) Complete immobilization to prevent injury
d) Use of a higher-pitched voice to ensure the patient can hear clearly

Answer: a) Greater reliance on verbal communication to convey information
Explanation: For patients with sensory disabilities such as blindness or low vision, greater reliance on verbal communication is essential to convey information and instructions. This ensures that the patient fully understands what is happening and can participate in their own care.

323. When providing emergency care to a patient with a mobility impairment, which of the following considerations should be prioritized?
a) The patient's comfort during transport
b) Ensuring proper immobilization of the affected limb or body part
c) The need for additional personnel or equipment to assist with moving the patient
d) All of the above

Answer: d) All of the above. Explanation: When providing emergency care to a patient with a mobility impairment, multiple considerations should be prioritized. This includes the patient's comfort during transport, ensuring proper immobilization of the affected limb or body part, and assessing the need for additional personnel or equipment to assist with moving the patient.

324. What is the key principle when providing emergency care to patients with disabilities?
a) Treat all patients with disabilities the same, regardless of their specific needs.
b) Focus on the disability rather than the patient's overall health and well-being.
c) Treat the patient with respect and dignity, adapting care to meet their unique needs.
d) Rely solely on the caregiver's input for decision-making and treatment.

Answer: c) Treat the patient with respect and dignity, adapting care to meet their unique needs. Explanation: The key principle when providing emergency care to patients with disabilities is to treat each patient with respect and dignity, adapting care to meet their unique needs. This includes focusing on the patient's overall health and well-being, rather than solely on their disability, and incorporating their perspective and preferences into decision-making and treatment.

325. Which of the following is a key component of cultural competence in emergency care?
a) Assuming all patients share the same beliefs and values
b) Relying on stereotypes to guide care decisions
c) Demonstrating empathy and understanding of a patient's cultural background
d) Ignoring the patient's cultural background to focus on their medical condition

Answer: c) Demonstrating empathy and understanding of a patient's cultural background
Explanation: Cultural competence in emergency care involves demonstrating empathy and understanding of a patient's cultural background, rather than relying on stereotypes or ignoring their background. This approach allows healthcare providers to better understand and respect patients' beliefs and values during treatment.

326. When providing emergency care to a patient from a different cultural background, it is essential to:
a) Insist on following the standard treatment protocol, regardless of cultural beliefs
b) Disregard the patient's wishes in favor of clinical best practices
c) Modify care based solely on the healthcare provider's assumptions about the patient's culture
d) Seek to understand and respect the patient's cultural beliefs and values

Answer: d) Seek to understand and respect the patient's cultural beliefs and values. Explanation: In order to provide culturally competent emergency care, healthcare providers should seek to understand and respect the patient's cultural beliefs and values. This approach allows for the adaptation of care when necessary and ensures that the patient's wishes and beliefs are respected during treatment.

327. Effective communication strategies for culturally competent emergency care include:
a) Speaking loudly and slowly to ensure the patient understands
b) Using medical jargon to convey information
c) Utilizing a professional interpreter when language barriers are present
d) Avoiding any discussion of cultural beliefs or values

Answer: c) Utilizing a professional interpreter when language barriers are present
Explanation: Effective communication is crucial in culturally competent emergency care. When language barriers are present, utilizing a professional interpreter can help ensure clear communication and understanding between the healthcare provider and the patient.

328. Cultural awareness in emergency care involves:
a) Assuming that all patients from the same cultural background have the same beliefs and values
b) Recognizing one's own biases and stereotypes
c) Ignoring cultural differences to focus on medical treatment
d) Believing that cultural differences do not impact patient care

Answer: b) Recognizing one's own biases and stereotypes
Explanation: Cultural awareness in emergency care involves recognizing one's own biases and stereotypes, as well as understanding how cultural differences can impact patient care. This awareness allows healthcare providers to adapt their approach to better meet the needs of diverse populations.

329. In order to provide culturally competent emergency care, healthcare providers should:
a) Focus solely on the patient's medical needs, disregarding their cultural background
b) Treat all patients the same, regardless of cultural differences
c) Adapt care to align with the patient's cultural beliefs and values, within the scope of clinical best practices
d) Assume that cultural beliefs and values do not impact emergency care

Answer: c) Adapt care to align with the patient's cultural beliefs and values, within the scope of clinical best practices
Explanation: Culturally competent emergency care involves adapting care to align with the patient's cultural beliefs and values, within the scope of clinical best practices. This approach respects the patient's cultural background while ensuring that appropriate medical care is provided.

330. Which of the following best describes the primary responsibility of an Emergency Medical Responder (EMR)?
a) Providing advanced life support interventions
b) Coordinating resources and scene management
c) Performing basic life support and initial patient assessment
d) Transporting patients to the appropriate healthcare facility

Answer: c) Performing basic life support and initial patient assessment
Explanation: The primary responsibility of an Emergency Medical Responder (EMR) is to perform basic life support and initial patient assessment. This role includes stabilizing the patient and providing essential care until more advanced medical personnel arrive.

331. Effective communication within an EMS team is crucial for:
a) Ensuring a fast response time
b) Improving the team's public image
c) Reducing the need for documentation
d) Coordinating patient care and maintaining patient safety

Answer: d) Coordinating patient care and maintaining patient safety
Explanation: Effective communication within an EMS team is crucial for coordinating patient care and maintaining patient safety. Clear communication allows for a better understanding of the patient's condition, treatment plan, and any potential complications, ensuring appropriate care is provided.

332. In an EMS system, the role of an Emergency Medical Technician (EMT) typically includes:
a) Providing only basic life support interventions
b) Performing advanced life support procedures
c) Assessing, treating, and transporting patients with a variety of medical and trauma-related conditions
d) Coordinating and directing the entire emergency response effort

Answer: c) Assessing, treating, and transporting patients with a variety of medical and trauma-related conditions
Explanation: The role of an Emergency Medical Technician (EMT) typically includes assessing, treating, and transporting patients with a variety of medical and trauma-related conditions. While EMTs are primarily focused on basic life support interventions, they may also assist with advanced life support procedures when necessary.

333. Which of the following best describes the role of a Paramedic within an EMS system?
a) Providing basic life support and initial patient assessment
b) Coordinating resources and scene management
c) Transporting patients to the appropriate healthcare facility
d) Performing advanced life support interventions and managing complex medical situations

Answer: d) Performing advanced life support interventions and managing complex medical situations
Explanation: The role of a Paramedic within an EMS system involves performing advanced life support interventions and managing complex medical situations. Paramedics have a higher level of training and expertise compared to EMTs, allowing them to provide more advanced care to patients.

334. The importance of collaboration among EMS team members is primarily to:
a) Reduce the workload for individual team members
b) Improve the team's reputation within the community
c) Enhance the overall effectiveness of patient care
d) Reduce the need for communication between team members

Answer: c) Enhance the overall effectiveness of patient care
Explanation: Collaboration among EMS team members is crucial for enhancing the overall effectiveness of patient care. Working together, team members can ensure that patients receive appropriate and timely treatment, leading to improved outcomes and a higher quality of care.

335. The primary role of an emergency medical dispatcher includes:
a) Providing medical treatment to patients over the phone
b) Coordinating and prioritizing emergency response resources
c) Transporting patients to the appropriate healthcare facility
d) Performing advanced life support interventions

Answer: b) Coordinating and prioritizing emergency response resources
Explanation: The primary role of an emergency medical dispatcher is to coordinate and prioritize emergency response resources. They are responsible for receiving incoming calls, gathering essential information, and dispatching appropriate EMS resources to the scene.

336. Which of the following is an essential component of call prioritization?
a) Ensuring a fast response time for all calls
b) Accurately assessing the severity of the situation
c) Maintaining a positive public image for the EMS system
d) Reducing the need for communication between team members

Answer: b) Accurately assessing the severity of the situation
Explanation: Accurately assessing the severity of the situation is an essential component of call prioritization. It allows emergency medical dispatchers to determine the appropriate level of response and allocate resources effectively.

337. The best practice for maintaining clear communication between EMS providers and dispatch centers is:
a) Using casual language to foster a relaxed atmosphere
b) Speaking quickly to convey information more efficiently
c) Utilizing standardized language and terminology
d) Relying on abbreviations and acronyms to save time

Answer: c) Utilizing standardized language and terminology
Explanation: Utilizing standardized language and terminology is the best practice for maintaining clear communication between EMS providers and dispatch centers. This approach ensures that all parties understand the information being conveyed, reducing the potential for miscommunication and errors.

338. When communicating with a receiving facility, EMS providers should prioritize:
a) Providing a comprehensive patient history
b) Discussing their personal assessment of the situation
c) Delivering a concise report, including critical information and interventions
d) Engaging in casual conversation to build rapport with hospital staff

Answer: c) Delivering a concise report, including critical information and interventions
Explanation: When communicating with a receiving facility, EMS providers should prioritize delivering a concise report, including critical information and interventions. This approach ensures that hospital staff have the necessary information to prepare for the patient's arrival and provide appropriate care.

339. The primary goal of effective communication in EMS is to:
a) Improve the efficiency of the EMS system
b) Reduce the need for documentation
c) Enhance patient care and safety
d) Foster camaraderie among team members

Answer: c) Enhance patient care and safety
Explanation: The primary goal of effective communication in EMS is to enhance patient care and safety. Clear and concise communication allows for a better understanding of the patient's condition, treatment plan, and any potential complications, ensuring appropriate care is provided.

340. Triage is a process that primarily focuses on:
a) Providing immediate medical care to all patients
b) Prioritizing patients based on the severity of their injuries
c) Transporting patients to the closest healthcare facility
d) Identifying and documenting all patients involved in the incident

Answer: b) Prioritizing patients based on the severity of their injuries
Explanation: Triage is a process that focuses on prioritizing patients based on the severity of their injuries. The goal of triage is to identify and treat the most critical patients first, maximizing the chances of survival for the largest number of people.

341. The START (Simple Triage and Rapid Treatment) system classifies patients into the following categories, except:
a) Immediate
b) Delayed
c) Minimal
d) Unresponsive

Answer: d) Unresponsive
Explanation: The START system classifies patients into Immediate, Delayed, and Minimal categories. The fourth category is Expectant, which includes patients who have injuries that are incompatible with life or require resources beyond what is available at the scene.

342. In a mass casualty incident, the primary responsibility of the incident commander is to:
a) Provide medical care to the most critically injured patients
b) Manage and coordinate the overall response effort
c) Act as the liaison between the public and the media
d) Assess and document the injuries of all patients

Answer: b) Manage and coordinate the overall response effort
Explanation: The primary responsibility of the incident commander in a mass casualty incident is to manage and coordinate the overall response effort. This includes directing resources, assigning tasks, and ensuring effective communication and collaboration among all responding agencies.

343. Which of the following is a key principle in managing mass casualty incidents?
a) Allocating resources equally among all patients
b) Providing the highest level of care possible to each individual patient
c) Focusing on the greatest good for the greatest number of people
d) Prioritizing patients based on their age and social status

Answer: c) Focusing on the greatest good for the greatest number of people
Explanation: In mass casualty incidents, the key principle is focusing on the greatest good for the greatest number of people. This means prioritizing resources and care based on the severity of injuries and the likelihood of survival, rather than trying to provide equal care to all patients.

344. The role of a medical branch director during a mass casualty incident includes:
a) Directly providing medical care to the most critically injured patients
b) Overseeing and coordinating all medical aspects of the response effort
c) Managing public relations and communication with the media
d) Ensuring the rapid transport of all patients to healthcare facilities

Answer: b) Overseeing and coordinating all medical aspects of the response effort
Explanation: The role of a medical branch director during a mass casualty incident is to oversee and coordinate all medical aspects of the response effort. This includes supervising medical personnel, managing triage and treatment areas, and coordinating the allocation of medical resources.

345. The primary purpose of the Incident Command System (ICS) is to:
a) Provide a standardized approach to emergency management
b) Delegate tasks to individual emergency responders
c) Organize emergency response resources by geographic location
d) Identify the most qualified personnel to serve in leadership roles

Answer: a) Provide a standardized approach to emergency management
Explanation: The primary purpose of the ICS is to provide a standardized approach to the command, control, and coordination of emergency response. It ensures a consistent framework for managing emergencies, regardless of their size or complexity.

346. Which of the following best describes the principle of "unity of command" within the ICS?
a) All responders report directly to the incident commander
b) Each responder reports to only one supervisor
c) Multiple agencies share command responsibilities
d) A single incident commander is responsible for all aspects of the response

Answer: b) Each responder reports to only one supervisor
Explanation: The principle of "unity of command" means that each responder reports to only one supervisor, ensuring a clear chain of command and reducing the potential for confusion or conflicting orders.

347. The Incident Command System is structured around five major functional areas, which include all of the following, except:
a) Command
b) Operations
c) Logistics
d) Intelligence

Answer: d) Intelligence
Explanation: The ICS is structured around five major functional areas: Command, Operations, Planning, Logistics, and Finance/Administration. Intelligence is not one of the five functional areas in the standard ICS structure.

348. In a large-scale incident requiring a multi-agency response, which ICS component is responsible for coordinating communication and resource allocation among the different agencies?
a) Incident Commander
b) Unified Command
c) Operations Section Chief
d) Public Information Officer

Answer: b) Unified Command
Explanation: In a large-scale incident requiring a multi-agency response, a Unified Command is established to coordinate communication and resource allocation among the different agencies involved. This ensures a collaborative approach to incident management while respecting the authority and jurisdiction of each agency.

349. The role of the Public Information Officer (PIO) within the ICS structure is to:
a) Serve as the incident commander's chief advisor
b) Coordinate the overall emergency response effort
c) Manage public relations and communication with the media and the public
d) Oversee resource allocation and logistics during the response

Answer: c) Manage public relations and communication with the media and the public
Explanation: The role of the Public Information Officer (PIO) within the ICS structure is to manage public relations and communication with the media and the public. The PIO is responsible for disseminating accurate and timely information about the incident and the response efforts, as well as addressing any rumors or misinformation that may arise.

350. Informed consent in EMS refers to:
a) Permission granted by a patient for treatment after they have been informed of the risks, benefits, and alternatives
b) Documenting a patient's medical history and treatment plan
c) Obtaining a patient's medical records from their primary care provider
d) Making medical decisions for a patient who is unconscious or unable to provide consent

Answer: a) Permission granted by a patient for treatment after they have been informed of the risks, benefits, and alternatives

Explanation: Informed consent is the process of obtaining permission from a patient to provide treatment after they have been informed of the risks, benefits, and alternatives. It is an essential part of patient care and ensures that patients have the right to make decisions about their healthcare.

351. When a patient refuses care or transportation against medical advice, it is important for EMS providers to:
a) Insist on providing care and transportation
b) Document the patient's refusal and ensure they understand the potential risks
c) Seek legal advice before continuing with treatment
d) Contact the patient's primary care provider for guidance

Answer: b) Document the patient's refusal and ensure they understand the potential risks

Explanation: When a patient refuses care or transportation against medical advice, EMS providers should document the patient's refusal and ensure they understand the potential risks associated with their decision. This helps protect both the patient and the EMS provider in case of legal issues.

352. The primary purpose of accurate and thorough documentation in EMS is to:
a) Protect the EMS provider from legal liability
b) Ensure proper billing for services provided
c) Provide a record of patient care for quality improvement and legal purposes
d) Communicate information about the patient's condition to other healthcare providers

Answer: c) Provide a record of patient care for quality improvement and legal purposes

Explanation: Accurate and thorough documentation in EMS serves to provide a record of patient care for quality improvement and legal purposes. It ensures continuity of care and helps protect both the patient and the EMS provider in case of legal issues.

353. When dealing with a minor who requires emergency care but whose parents or legal guardians are not present, EMS providers should:
a) Wait for the parents or legal guardians to arrive before providing care
b) Obtain consent from another adult present at the scene
c) Provide care under the principle of implied consent
d) Contact the patient's primary care provider for guidance

Answer: c) Provide care under the principle of implied consent

Explanation: When dealing with a minor who requires emergency care but whose parents or legal guardians are not present, EMS providers should provide care under the principle of implied consent. Implied consent assumes that the patient or their legal guardian would consent to treatment if they were able to do so.

354. The principle of patient confidentiality in EMS means that:
a) EMS providers must obtain consent from the patient before sharing their information with other healthcare providers
b) EMS providers cannot disclose patient information to anyone outside of their EMS agency
c) EMS providers can share patient information with anyone who is directly involved in the patient's care
d) EMS providers should not discuss patient information in public or share it with unauthorized individuals

Answer: d) EMS providers should not discuss patient information in public or share it with unauthorized individuals

Explanation: The principle of patient confidentiality in EMS means that EMS providers should not discuss patient information in public or share it with unauthorized individuals. Patient information should only be shared with those directly involved in the patient's care or as required by law.

In conclusion, the CFRN exam represents a significant milestone in your journey to excel in the critical care and emergency nursing field. This study guide has been meticulously crafted to support and encourage you throughout the learning process, covering a wide array of crucial topics that you will encounter on the exam. We understand that this experience might have included moments of uncertainty and difficulty, but always remember that every challenge you face ultimately contributes to your professional growth and development.

Throughout this study guide, we have delved into essential subjects such as temperature-related emergencies, drowning and near-drowning incidents, animal bites and stings, high altitude emergencies, traumatic injuries, pediatric and geriatric emergencies, obstetric and gynecological emergencies, mental health crisis management, emergency care for patients with disabilities, cultural competence, roles and responsibilities within EMS, communication in EMS, principles of triage, the Incident Command System, and legal and ethical considerations in EMS operations. As you move forward, use your past experiences to learn and grow, transforming you into a more empathetic and skilled healthcare professional.

This comprehensive study guide has been designed to mitigate your fears by presenting the material in an organized, succinct, and approachable manner, empowering you to face the exam with self-assurance. We recognize that the CFRN exam may validate some of your suspicions about the intricacy and depth of critical care and emergency nursing, but rest assured that this study guide lays a strong foundation of knowledge, providing you with the tools to overcome any hurdles along the way.

Lastly, we are committed to supporting you in your pursuit of greatness. We stand with you as you confront the challenges of the CFRN exam and your future career, offering guidance and encouragement whenever required. With determination, persistence, and a reliable support system, you are well-prepared to tackle the CFRN exam and achieve your goals in the world of critical care and emergency nursing.